Short-Term Psychodynamic Psychotherapy

Alan Eppel

Short-Term Psychodynamic Psychotherapy

Springer

Alan Eppel
McMaster University
Hamilton
Ontario
Canada

ISBN 978-3-030-09123-1 ISBN 978-3-319-74995-2 (eBook)
https://doi.org/10.1007/978-3-319-74995-2

Softcover re-print of the Hardcover 1st edition 2018

Printed on acid-free paper
This Springer imprint is published by the registered company Springer International Publishing AG part of Springer Nature
The registered company address is: Gewerbestrasse 11, 6330 Cham, Switzerland

Preface

It was in the spring of 1976 that I travelled from Union Station in Toronto to the Gare Centrale, Montreal's central train station at the Queen Elizabeth Hotel. The occasion was an international conference organized by Habib Davanloo on short-term psychodynamic psychotherapy. At the time I was a resident in psychiatry at McMaster University in Hamilton Ontario. Short-term psychodynamic psychotherapy was still very new in the wider psychotherapeutic and psychiatric universes.

The conference brought together the leading pioneers in the field: Peter Sifneos, David Malan and of course Davanloo himself.

The conference was a thrilling experience because the presenters showed videotapes of themselves in sessions with real patients. This allowed the conference participants to test the well-known clinical adage that what psychotherapists think they do and what they actually do are not always a match. In Montreal we had the astounding opportunity to watch these experts at work and see for ourselves.

I later learned that Malan was so impressed with Davanloo's technique that he modified his own approach and subsequently collaborated with Davanloo.

Sifneos described his short-term anxiety provoking psychotherapy, STAP, which he was developing at Massachusetts General and Beth Israel Hospital in Boston. Sifneos would identify a circumscribed specific chief complaint in order to reach agreement with the patient on one problem. A requirement for his therapy was that the patient had had at least one meaningful relationship during his life, a relationship characterized by give and take, some flexibility and some altruism.

The patient also needed to demonstrate an ability to interact with the therapist in a flexible way. Motivation for change was another requirement for acceptance into STAP. Sifneos practised a focal model of psychotherapy. His technique involved raising the level of anxiety in the session to an optimal level in order to reduce defenses and facilitate expression.

David Malan also had adopted a focal conflict methodology and a systematic approach to patient evaluation and therapeutic interventions.

None of this could prepare the audience for Habib Davanloo. The impact for many was one of shock. Davanloo's forceful confrontational style was a dramatic change from the more gentle and obviously empathetic approaches of the other therapists.

Davanloo's approach was powerful and implicitly conveyed empathy by the intensity of his commitment to breaking through the defenses.

At the time my own supervisors at McMaster had very different styles. Dr. Nahum Spinner used what might be termed a narrative approach. He would illustrate central concepts by anecdotes and stories about his colleagues or himself. These stories had in reality the qualities of a parable illustrating important therapeutic principles laced with strong doses of compassion. He rarely used technical jargon. As a first year resident this puzzled me as I did not know what I was learning. In retrospect Dr. Spinner exemplified what is now called a relational approach, an approach infused with a profound humanism and an existential sensibility. He captured the essence of psychotherapy in situating the process in the "you-me domain". This had echoes with Martin Buber's famous treatise on "I and thou".

Another of my supervisors, Jock Cleghorn, had trained as a psychoanalyst but was also interested in the neuroscience of sleep. Jock was the first to introduce me to the focal conflict model based on the work of Thomas French. Conflicts were identified between a disturbing wish or need and a reactive motive.

Over the following three decades of practising general psychiatry in busy inpatient and outpatient settings, I learned much about the importance of attachment in human relationships. This arose from treating patients with borderline personality disorder. It was clear that a central feature of these patients' difficulty was insecure attachment with avoidant and preoccupied patterns. The attachment model seemed much more relevant than the theories of the day.

In 2000 after returning to McMaster University I began to supervise psychiatry residents in psychodynamic psychotherapy. I thought it would be useful to acquire one of Davanloo's videotapes to show to the residents. No tapes were publicly available. However in my Google searches I stumbled upon a DVD produced by Diana Fosha, a psychologist working in New York City.

I ordered this DVD. My first impression was to dismiss it as it seemed so radically different from anything I had seen before. However the more I watched, the more I was stunned by the complexity and at the same time simplicity of her approach and its dramatic impact.

Fosha had turned Davanloo's method "on its head" while maintaining the fundamental principles of dynamic psychotherapy. She described her therapy as "accelerated", and its effects were evident right from the opening gambits.

I had to get more of this approach and subsequently attended AEDP courses and supervision with Eileen Russell in New York.

Diana Fosha's approach dramatically changed my own approach to therapy. The emphasis was now on affect much more than intellectual insight.

I was anxious to convey these dramatically improved approaches to residents in supervision.

In the course of supervising residents it became apparent that experienced therapists were able to choose different interventions than beginners. This provoked the recollection of an educational session I had attended as a resident in psychiatry presented by Lewis Tauber. Tauber was a group psychotherapist and supervised group, individual and family psychotherapy at McMaster University in Hamilton Ontario. He had introduced us to the concept of "choice points" in group therapy. I found my old notes and was able to track down his original 1978 paper online. I felt that it was a brilliant tool that could be expanded to enhance the supervision of residents. I began to use it in the following years. I was able to communicate by email with Dr. Tauber, and I am glad to say that he was pleased to hear that his method was again being used for supervising learners.

Ultimately my experience with this approach led me to consider writing a manual for residents that subsequently evolved into the writing of this book.

What is the place of short-term psychodynamic psychotherapy in current-day clinical practice? After six decades the promise of the psychopharmacological revolution has been only partially realized. Perhaps our expectations were naïve. Medications while powerful and effective in reducing symptoms cannot be expected to address critical emotional and personal dimensions of illness. Medications belong to a class of therapeutics that is directed at symptom elimination. On its own it comprises only one part of the biopsychosocial triangle. The use of medications mechanistically results in the loss of the essential person-to-person healing relationship.

Access to psychotherapy services remains unequal to the needs of patients. The methods and level of funding for psychotherapeutic services vary quite considerably from country to country, e.g. in North America, Europe and Australia. There is a need for effective short-term psychotherapies. Cognitive behaviour therapy has a well-established role in clinical practice and has often displaced psychodynamic approaches because of its shorter lengths of treatment. However cognitive behaviour therapy and related approaches are not effective for all patients, and a broader array of therapy options needs to be available to patients.

Over the past two decades a significant evidence base has been accumulating to demonstrate that short-term psychodynamic psychotherapy can achieve good treatment outcomes. A manualized approach can lead to more effective therapy implementation and outcomes. Manuals can enhance the training of supervisees and facilitate research studies.

I should stress here what probably is quite obvious: one cannot become a psychotherapist by learning from textbooks or manuals. The essence of psychotherapy is the experience of the therapeutic relationship and using that to alleviate suffering. Descriptions on the written page do not convey the emotional intensity, the connection between patient and therapist and the dynamic flow of psychotherapy.

This book describes concepts from neuroscience, attachment theory and decision theory. These disciplines constitute foundational knowledge for the practice of psychotherapy. The other sections of the book elaborate the conduct of therapy drawing on research findings and the deployment of specific skills. Psychodynamic psychotherapy cannot be done in a mechanical way. However this book allows therapists to acquire a model that contains enough definition to produce a consistent approach. At the same time it retains a flexibility that allows for moments of spontaneity and creativity.

This book is unique in a number of ways:

- It is not based on a specific school of psychoanalytic or psychodynamic theory. Rather I have attempted to extract and integrate key concepts.
- It attempts to move away from language that is derived from theories and concepts that have been superseded by advances in psychology and neuroscience.
- It provides definitions of concepts that are more in keeping with scientific understanding as opposed to their metaphorical origins.

Description of This Book

Chapters 1, 2, 3, 4, 5 and 6 cover the theoretical underpinnings of the practice of STPP. Chapter 1 describes the evolution of the short-term psychodynamic psychotherapies starting in Europe in the 1920s. Chapter 2 on attachment theory provides a framework for understanding adult relationship patterns and internal working models.

Chapter 3 reviews the nature of emotions beginning with Darwin's momentous observations and then moving forward to our current understanding of the dual system model of emotion processing. This chapter reviews the complex relationships between consciousness and the subcortical origins of emotions. This knowledge base has direct applicability to the change process in STPP. Therapists must be able to recognize, elicit and process emotion. This is essential for the practice of short-term psychodynamic therapy (STPP).

Chapter 4 is a brief but critical overview of the research literature on short-term psychodynamic therapy.

Chapter 5 discusses the language of psychodynamic psychotherapy and proposes neuroscientific updates in redefining these fundamental concepts.

Chapter 6 expands on Tauber's ideas and describes one of the unique features of this book: "Choice Point Analysis" and "Action Alternatives" which facilitate the practice and the supervision of psychodynamic psychotherapy. The evidence linking key interventions with clinical outcomes is reviewed.

Chapter 7 essentially forms a manual that describes the objectives, tasks and methods for conducting short-term dynamic psychotherapy across the phases of Engagement, Emotion Processing and Termination. The Engagement phase covers the establishment of the therapeutic alliance and the beginnings of therapy. The Emotion-Processing phase involves working with the therapeutic relationship, the relational focus and processing affect.

Chapter 8 demonstrates how the manual can be applied to the supervision of trainees and contains extracts of a case transcript which has been annotated to demonstrate the choice point method.

The concepts and interventions described in this book have great utility in a wide range of practice settings. There is much benefit in adopting a psychodynamically informed approach to general clinical work.

Chapter 9 describes the application of STPP principles to general clinical practice. This is for physicians, psychologists, social worker and others who may not be in a position to undertake systematic psychotherapy. Throughout the emphasis is on clarity, succinctness and easy readability.

A Note About Terminology

There are numerous variations of psychodynamic psychotherapy. Many of these are considered to fall under the umbrella of short-term psychodynamic psychotherapy because they embrace the major concepts and approaches which are reflected in this publication. The terms "experiential dynamic psychotherapy" and "supportive-expressive psychodynamic psychotherapy" are used to describe these same approaches. The goal has been to avoid non-generic jargon and use terminology that is applicable and common across the disciplines.

This book does not follow one specific school of psychodynamic psychotherapy. It is an integrated model and contains elements from many of the leaders in the field. It is based on a focal approach and incorporates experiential, emotion-based and relational interventions.

I have highlighted the implications of research findings that show that expert clinicians make use of intuition and experience. This manifests in a level of spontaneity in the kinds of interventions made by experts. I became very much aware of this in watching Nate Epstein make rapid assessments of complex family dynamics. He used intuition and skills that were invisible to myself and other psychiatry residents. Trainees and early career psychotherapists do not have this hidden repertoire to draw upon. For a student of psychodynamic psychotherapy the task at times seems overwhelming. Choice Point Analysis and the selection of Action Alternatives are central to this book in order to make the learning process more effective. It may potentially open up a new dimension to psychotherapy training, practice and research.

I would like to acknowledge those who influenced me along the way. This includes the hundreds of patients I have treated over the years who have impacted on my own self-concept and ways of relating and my supervisors Nahum Spinner, Jock Cleghorn, Wendall Waters, Ron Ruskin, Emile Zamora and Gian Bartolucci. A particular thanks to Nate Epstein, founding chairman of the Department of Psychiatry at McMaster University and brilliant family therapist, for setting the events in motion that shaped my own trajectory leading to arrival at this destination. I must recognize my resident supervisees who provided inspiration as we grappled with the art and science of psychotherapy. To Elaine Chow and Yu Jiang thank you for your assistance.

Gratitude and kudos to Diana Fosha, Eileen Russell and others in the AEDP community for their transforming influence.

I would like to express appreciation to David Abrahamson who has provided important advice and ideas since my entry into psychiatry. His incisive intellect and clarity of reasoning have been of great value to me. His work as a psychiatrist in the National Health Service in the UK has been an inspiration in demonstrating integrity and a total commitment to improving the lives of patients.

To James Bourgeois for his guidance and generous support. To Ana Hategan for her insights and encouragement to complete this volume in her inimitable frank and direct way. To Randi McCabe for her expert advice on developing psychotherapy manuals.

To Molly Ferguson who has done a superb job of creating delightful illustrations of emotions.

And finally to Nadina Persaud and Prakash Jagannathan at Springer for their patient assistance and advice.

Canada
December 2017

Alan Eppel

Contents

Chapter 1
The Emergence of Short-Term Psychodynamic Psychotherapy

1.1 Origins

We must look to Budapest Hungary in order to trace the origins of STPP. It is there in the persona of Sandor Ferenczi that Freud's treatment parameters were challenged. Ferenczi began to experiment with a more active approach [1]. He put a greater emphasis on emotion as opposed to interpretation. Another Hungarian and an analysand of Ferenczi, Franz Alexander was also to figure prominently in the elaboration of shorter and more focused interventions.

Alexander and French in 1946 introduced the idea of the "corrective emotional experience" [2, 3]. This idea was initially rebuffed by mainstream practitioners. However it can now be seen as a forerunner of the current emphasis on the relationship aspects of psychotherapy as opposed to interpretation.

Alexander's identification of the corrective emotional experience was an important break with the emphasis on interpretation as the curative vehicle. Corrective emotional experiences depend on a strong therapeutic alliance with the therapist, emotional expression and disconfirmation of the patients' feared expectations. Reflecting on the experience, the self-reflective loop is essential for the therapeutic impact. This is what distinguishes the corrective emotional experience from mere catharsis which is not effective.

A. Eppel, *Short-Term Psychodynamic Psychotherapy*,
https://doi.org/10.1007/978-3-319-74995-2_1

Sandor Ferenczi and the Budapest School are now recognized for introducing major technical shifts that gave rise to more active interventions emphasizing what are now regarded as "relational" interventions. Ferenczi diverged from Freud in the focus on the interactions between patient and therapist.

Alice and Michael Balint, disciples of Ferenczi, moved to London England from Hungary and had a profound impact on the outlook of the Independent School of British Object Relations in particular on Winnicott, Malan and Bowlby [4–13]. Balint had translated Ferenczi's work into English. Balint and Winnicott's therapeutic styles provide the conceptual links between object relations theory and Bowlby's attachment theory (Fig. 1.1).

At the Tavistock clinic in London, Balint influenced and worked closely with David Malan. Malan by introducing a dynamic focus and attention to transference interpretations can be regarded as one of the founding fathers of the modern-day short-term dynamic approaches [3–9].

I have illustrated the relationships between these psychoanalysts and psychotherapists in the adjoining figures. The connecting lines are to indicate influence on theory and practice. These connections are based on my own readings and may not necessarily be accepted by the authors themselves.

The work of Michael Balint and David Malan marks a critical point in the breakout of short-term dynamic psychotherapy. Balint was a starkly creative and original psychotherapist.

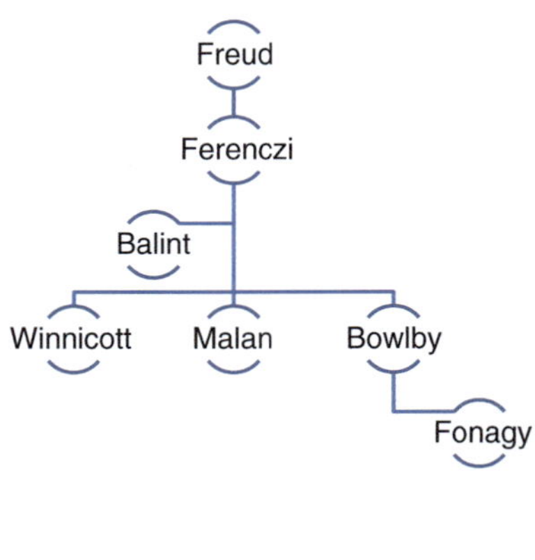

Figure 1.1 Major contributors to the development of STPP

It is to Balint that we attribute the concept of "focal psychotherapy". His approach while deeply rooted in Freudian ideas of impulses and defence also contains a revolutionary interpersonal perspective. This was evident in his 1957 book *The Doctor, His Patient and The Illness*. In this he conceives illness as an interpersonal construct [10].

We normally think of illness as something that is contained within the body of the patient. But Balint brings attention to focus on the interpersonal dimensions of illness behaviour and the interactions that ensue between the patient and physician. The patient "offers" symptoms and complaints, and the physician makes a counteroffer. This is a constructivist view long before such ideas became popular and recognized as such. The patient and the physician co-construct the illness. Counteroffers could be in the form of investigations or medications. In addition for Balint a counteroffer could consist of listening deeply, "being with" and staying with the patient through his difficulties. This was quite a radical way to view the physician's task. Balint proposed that the doctor him or herself could be the offering and could take the place of medication and be administered in different "dosages". This foreshadowed the current emphasis on the relationship in psychodynamic therapy.

Balint like Winnicott was intensely aware of the nonverbal and relational dimensions and that the way of relating itself could be therapeutic. For Malan interpretation dominated the therapeutic approach until his encounter with Davanloo.

In 1963, Malan published his first book demonstrating focal psychotherapy [6]. He named his approach "brief psychotherapy" and underlined the importance of interpreting the transference.

Malan wanted to put psychoanalytic treatment on a scientific basis and to make it more accessible by shortening the process. He worked on developing selection criteria, therapeutic strategies and measures of outcome.

Malan discovered that it was possible to make radical interpretations of the transference and that this was associated with better results. Malan made use of the parallels in the patient's past relationships, current relationships and transference relationship. He referred to this as the "triangle of conflict". In a subsequent study, Malan found that positive outcome was related to the percentage of parent-transference links made by the therapist. This finding would turn out to be not so straightforward in research conducted in later decades (Chap. 4).

At this early stage, Malan held that the strategic aim of brief psychotherapy was to bring emotional conflicts into consciousness. The focus on a single conflict differentiated brief psychotherapy from classical psychoanalysis.

1.2 The Triangles

Malan used diagrams of triangles to systematically conceptualize some of the key activities required of the therapist in psychodynamic psychotherapy.

The origins of this approach are derived from the concept of "working through" [14]. Working through refers to repeated interpretations in order to promote insight.

Karl Menninger had described the "triangle of insight" as a framework for working through [15]. This involves identifying transference patterns and relating them to patterns in current and developmental relationships. Malan elaborated on these ideas and named this "the triangle of the person" (Fig. 1.2).

The first corner of the triangle represents current relationships, the second corner represents past relationships, and the third corner represents the transference. The triangular representation reinforces the idea that the same relationship pattern may be evident in past, present and therapeutic relationships.

Henry Ezriel, a group psychotherapist also working at the Tavistock in London England, further developed and structured the use of transference interpretations.

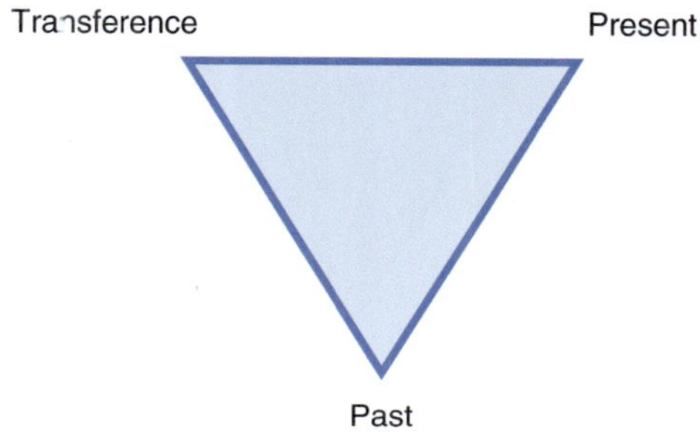

FIGURE 1.2 Triangle of the Person

Ezriel made a huge conceptual leap which presages the whole relational movement in psychodynamic psychotherapy. He recognized that although transference patterns are derived from past relationships, they are operative in the here-and-now present moment [16].

Ezriel focused on the therapist-patient relationship. He described the patient's need to relate to the therapist in a particular way which he called the "required relationship". He also identified "the avoided relationship" which was a type of relationship that the patient unconsciously wanted to avoid. This feared relationship was based on the unconscious expectation that it could lead to a "calamitous" outcome. The feared or calamitous outcome is the result of giving in to the desire of entering into the avoided relationship.

Malan based his triangle of conflict on similar ideas (Fig. 1.3). Ezriel's required relationship is equivalent to Malan's defences, the avoided relationship to the wish and anxiety to the feared outcome.

The major advance that Ezriel made was to distinguish what had occurred in the past from the activity in the present. He highlighted that transference is not something that gradually develops in the course of therapy but that it is active from the very first meeting between the patient and therapist [15]. Transference is an expectation, a prediction of how our relationships will play out. It can also be viewed as an attempt to

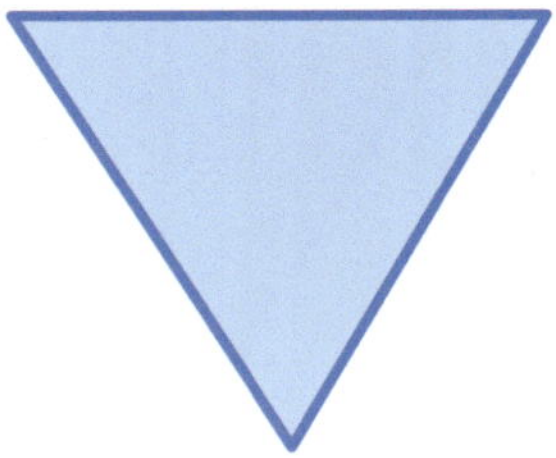

FIGURE 1.3 Triangle of conflict

establish or re-create in the here and now a particular relationship pattern. Ezriel goes on to say:

> This means that everything the patient says or does during the session – movements, gestures, phantasies, dreams, and even deliberate lies – is considered as the *idiom* used by the patient to give expression to his need in that session for a specific relationship with his therapist [15].

Malan initially maintained the belief that interpretation was the most important component of the therapeutic process. In contrast his mentor Michael Balint felt that the quality and nature of the therapeutic relationship was critical to successful therapy.

After studying Davanloo's methods and results, Malan came to the conclusion that his prior work at the Tavistock Clinic based mainly on an interpretive approach was "inadequate" [5, 7, 8]. And in fact interpretations might get in the way of allowing the patient to experience his feelings [5]. Malan came to the conclusion that a new approach was required and believed that Davanloo's methods provided some of the essential components for changes in practice [7, 8].

Malan was now convinced that dealing with emotion was more important than making interpretations. The strategy in therapy now becomes getting to the feelings and facilitating the patient's deep experience of these emotions.

1.3 The Meaning of Time: James Mann

James Mann was one of the few authors who has grappled with the unstated and implicit components within short-term psychodynamic therapies, the concept and meaning of time [16, 17].

Mann worked at the Boston University School of Medicine and Medical Center. In 1964, faced with long waiting lists and heavy demands for service, Mann introduced a time-limited method of psychotherapy. He implemented a general policy within his clinic that all patients would be offered 12 treatment hours.

Mann deliberately employed time to achieve the goals of therapy. The choice of 12 treatment sessions was arbitrary, but Mann felt that this was the minimal time required for resolution.

Mann used a focal conflict approach identifying a recurrent issue that has led to maladaptive functioning. To emphasize the importance of time in his approach, the patient was given the times for each appointment as well as the exact date of the 12th and final session. This was to prevent the patient from avoiding thoughts about the ending of therapy and its associated separation anxiety. Mann described his approach as designed to overcome the unconscious yearnings for the timelessness experienced in childhood in relation to the mother [16].

1.4 Emotional Crisis and Grief: Erich Lindemann, Peter Sifneos and Habib Davanloo

Less widely discussed today is the very significant impact that Erich Lindemann had on the current practice of short-term dynamic psychotherapies through two of his psychiatry residents, Peter Sifneos and Habib Davanloo.

Lindemann developed a rapid therapeutic approach to individuals experiencing grief and loss following a nightclub fire in 1945. Lindemann noticed that rapid psychological change could occur following a major trauma. The trauma of death often resulted in a breakdown of the normal defensive barriers and resistance to psychological change. The patient's mental state was more "fluid" and amenable to change [18].

Lindemann's approach to grief involved that the patient focus on both positive and negative feelings towards the deceased person. The patient needed to become aware of psychological factors that blocked the experience of grief in order to experience the emotional pain of bereavement rather than avoiding it. His ideas appear to have had an important influence on Sifneos and Davanloo [19–23].

Davanloo applied some of these principles to psychotherapy in general [21, 22]. To do this it meant re-creating some of the same conditions of psychological flexibility in order to lead to rapid intrapsychic change. The method he developed was to vigorously confront, to create pressure by focusing intensely on the transference in order to break through to unconscious material. Davanloo was also one of the first to use videotaped recordings of sessions for teaching and supervision but also for research. Davanloo called his approach "Intensive Short-Term Dynamic Psychotherapy", and his method is widely practised and taught in Halifax Nova Scotia, California and elsewhere in the United States, the Netherlands, Norway, Sweden and the United Kingdom.

Davanloo moved to McGill University in Montréal in the 1960s where he developed and refined his techniques. Davanloo's method is intensely experiential facilitating and amplifying the patient's experience of emotion which allows for a reworking of the patient's perception of himself and others. The emphasis is on the immediate experience within the therapeutic session with particular attention to the patient's feelings and emotions towards the therapist.

Davanloo's technique represented a further leap in the evolution of short-term psychodynamic psychotherapy. Davanloo's students went on to branch out and expand this method.

Davanloo and Sifneos recognized that therapy could be facilitated by deliberately manipulating the level of anxiety. Sifneos called his method "short-term anxiety-provoking psychotherapy" [20, 21]. It is well established that there is an optimal level of anxiety needed to facilitate the learning process, so too is this the case with psychotherapy.

Davanloo's approach takes this a step further by deliberately raising the temperature and increasing the level of tension in order to break down the defences to get to the underlying emotions at the bottom of the triangle of conflict.

This involves a period of "pressure" in which the therapist identifies contradictions and inconsistencies. Defences are challenged. This involves very active intervention by the therapist often interrupting. This in turn intensifies emotional arousal and feelings of anger.

This activates transference feelings and resistance. These feelings contain a mixture of anger, sadness, loss and longings for intimacy. At the same time, the therapist conveys that this challenging of defences is necessary for the patient's recovery and to relieve his suffering. The therapy proceeds working with cycles of defence, challenge and transference.

Challenge to the resistance in the transference eventually results in a breakthrough with the expression of unconscious feelings and memories. Davanloo referred to this breakthrough as "unlocking the unconscious".

This phase facilitates the exploration of outside relationship patterns and again working through cycles of defence and emotion. This is an iterative process in which relationships are explored and new resistances are addressed with further challenge.

Interpretations are made linking the resistance in the transference with conflicts in both current and past relationships utilising the three corners of the triangle of the person: transference-current-past, in short "TCP interpretations" [7, 8].

In the history of psychodynamic psychotherapy, perhaps there has never been such an abrupt and transformational change in practice and technique.

For those in the early 1970s who viewed Davanloo's video recordings, the impact was dramatic. For many this radical change was shocking and antithetical to the more gradualist and long-term approach that cut across mainstream psychodynamic psychotherapy. Davanloo's techniques elicited intense emotion in the here and now of the therapeutic session. This is the basis of the experiential approach.

Despite the objections and repudiation by traditional psychoanalysts, Davanloo's approach was in its essence a distillation of psychodynamic tenets. He followed the basic sequence of identifying defences and getting past these to unconscious material. He made amplified use of the transference to accelerate and intensify the process but at the same time mobilized and strengthened the unconscious therapeutic alliance.

1.5 Manualized Psychotherapy: Lester Luborsky

Lester Luborsky trained and worked at the Menninger Foundation and then with a group of researchers in Pennsylvania where he developed his core conflictual relationship theme approach [24]. This was a manual-based approach for identifying a core transference theme. He used audio recordings of patient interviews and specific rating scales (Fig. 1.4).

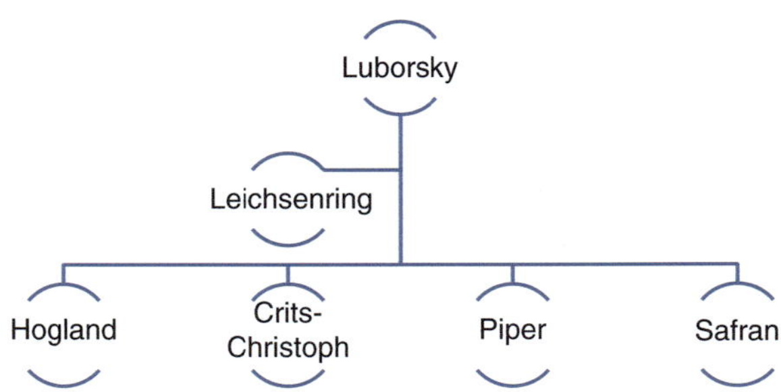

FIGURE 1.4 Second-generation researchers in STPP

He described his approach As Supportive Expressive Psychoanalytically Oriented Psychotherapy based on the model practised at the Menninger. Supportive techniques are those that enhance and support the therapeutic relationship. Expressive techniques are those that facilitate the expressions of feelings, thoughts and reflection leading to insight or understanding. Expressive techniques aim to supply meaning to what the patient expresses.

Luborsky defined a time-limited version of his approach named as "SE-TL". This time-limited version lasted from 6 to 25 sessions with a session frequency of once or twice per week. He described that his time-limited therapy is "in the lineage of short-term psychotherapies" which includes Balint, Malan, Sifneos and Mann [24].

Like these other authors, Luborsky adopts a consistent therapeutic focus. This involves making a selection early in the treatment of a primary focus around which the therapy will be directed. The focus is usually based on a component of the core conflictual relationship theme and the symptoms connected with it [24].

The core conflictual relationship theme consists of:

- A wish, need or intention – W
- An executive function which appraises the likely impact of acting on the wish, need or intention
- The responses from the other person – RO
- The responses of the self

The task of the therapist is to help the patient achieve insight by working through the multiple examples of the relationship theme as they are expressed in the transference. This involves dealing with the defence "resistances" that block the emergence into awareness of unconscious thoughts and feelings [24]. Examples of wishes include to be assertive, to feel strong or to be independent. Response from the object could be in the form of domination, intrusion, rejection, or disapproval. Positive responses would be acceptance and caring. Responses from the self may consist of withdrawal, passively going along, anger or anxiety.

1.6 The Third Generation of STPPs

Davanloo had a profound influence on three of his students: Allan Abbass, Diana Fosha and Leigh McCullough who went on to elaborate or modify his methods (Fig. 1.5).

There is considerable overlap in the work of these three master therapists (Figs. 1.6 and 1.7).

1.6.1 Allan Abbass

Allan Abbass completed a family practice residency at McGill University in Montréal. He worked as a family and emergency physician. He started training with Davanloo in 1990 and subsequently completed psychiatry residency training in Toronto. He continued to practise the Davanloo model

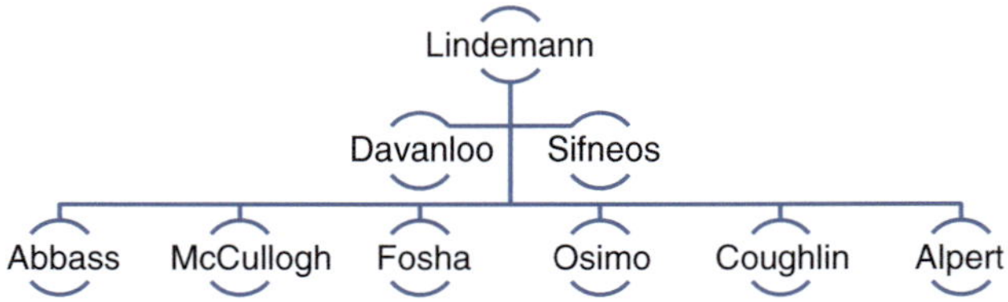

FIGURE 1.5 The third generation of STPPs

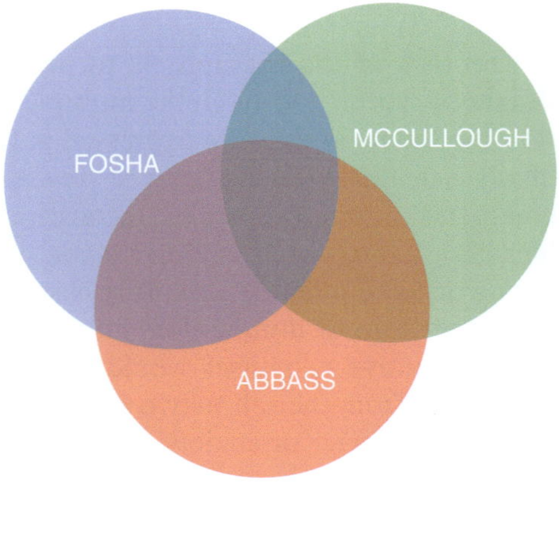

FIGURE 1.6 Relationship of third-generation STPP to each other

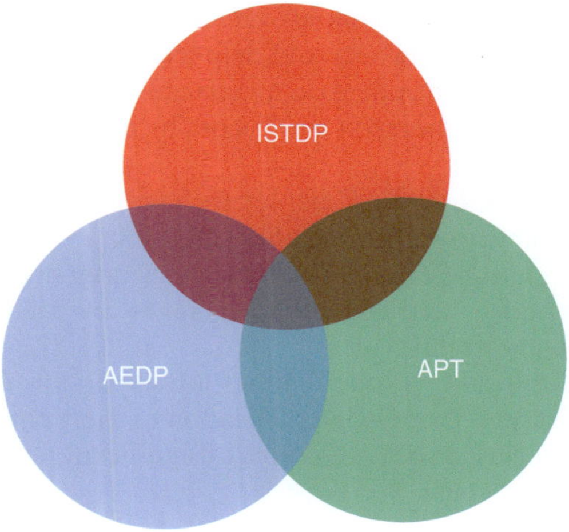

FIGURE 1.7 Experiential dynamic psychotherapies

and set up a training centre at Dalhousie University in Nova Scotia. He has provided training internationally and has been a prolific researcher publishing multiple empirical studies of ISTDP [25–28]. He has demonstrated the economic benefits of treating psychosomatic disorders with ISTDP.

In his more recent publications, Abbass and his colleagues in Sweden have replaced the term "unlocking the unconscious" with "mobilization of unprocessed complex emotions" (MUCE) [29]. Therapy is conceptualized as mobilizing and processing these emotions. This change of terminology is welcomed as it relinquishes historical terms and introduces those that have been enriched by advances in neuroscience and emotion theory. The change in terminology also facilitates more compatibility of language between ISTDP and other forms of emotion-focused experiential treatment.

ISTDP recognizes three levels of emotional arousal and expressiveness:

- Low rise in which there is little emotional activation and the dialogue is intellectual Defences and anxiety are minimally apparent.

- High rise in which complex attachment-related emotions are evident with anxiety and defences. These defences are distancing and include gaze avoidance, turning of the body away from the therapist and becoming more passive in the interview.
- Partial breakthrough. Complex feelings are at a high level. The patient experiences feelings of grief.
- Partial unlocking. Patient now experiences deep feelings such as grief, rage and guilt. Linkages are made to past attachment trauma.
- Major unlocking strong feelings are experienced towards the therapist. There is intensification of the treatment alliance associated with memories of significant persons from the patient's past.

1.6.2 Affect Phobia Therapy: Leigh McCullough

Affect phobia therapy was developed by Leigh McCullough [30]. She began research on short-term dynamic psychotherapy in the 1980s at the Beth Israel Medical Center in New York.

She later became director of the Psychotherapy Research Program at Harvard Medical School. Her work has been continued since her death by Kristin Osborn and Nathaniel Kuhn.

Her intensive review of videotape sessions led her to reformulate the process of therapy. She identified that the fear of experiencing emotions is central to the development of patients' difficulties [30–32]. She incorporated aspects of learning theory and cognitive behaviour therapy into her model. She felt that fear of affect which she entitled "affect phobia" was analogous to external phobias such as agoraphobia in which the main coping strategy was avoidance. She applied the same principles of APT treatment that involved gradual desensitization to the experience of painful emotions. She viewed her therapy as an integration of dynamic and behavioural principles.

Defences represent avoidance strategies. These include withdrawal, avoiding eye contact, smiling when talking about something sad, changing the subject, focusing on physical symptoms and self-criticism.

APT works with defences which are used to avoid the experience of uncomfortable feelings or to maintain them out of awareness. The principal shift in this form of STPP is the reconceptualization using concepts from learning theory and behaviour therapy, i.e. avoidance and the need for exposure. She also included the use of guided imagery to elicit memories and sensations connected to painful emotions. The therapeutic process is modelled on systematic desensitization from learning theory. This involves exposure to the feared emotion and response prevention by means of discouraging avoidance of emotions. The gradual exposure to these emotions within the context of an empathic therapeutic relationship fosters healing.

The work of McCullough's group has involved meticulous analysis of videotapes broken down into 10-min segments. Affect phobias frequently involve feelings of grief, anger, assertiveness, sexuality, aggression, closeness and positive feelings towards the self [30, 31]. These are considered adaptive or activating affects. Anxiety and shame are considered inhibitory affects.

Activating affects lead to activity, approach, engagement and opening up. Inhibitory affects lead to withdrawal, avoidance and shutting down.

Affect phobia therapy also makes use of the triangle of conflict. There is a focus on the impact of inhibitory affects and defences that block the experience of conflict between adaptive affects and inhibitory affects.

Treatment is accomplished by means of helping the patient experience more adaptive affect in a gradual way while attenuating feelings of anxiety, shame and guilt. Affects are considered as the primary motivators of behaviour. The experience of affect is fundamental to therapeutic change.

Affect phobia therapy utilizes graded exposure to the feared emotion. Over the course of therapy, the patient is able to tolerate the experience of increasing levels of the feared affect. The patient is encouraged to stay with his or her feelings.

Anxiety regulation is another component of AFP. This involves ensuring that the anxiety level is not too high. If the anxiety levels are not modulated, there is a risk of having the reverse of the intended effect by increasing the sensitization to the feared affect.

The goal is to free up the inner experience of adaptive emotions by breaking "the stranglehold that anxiety, guilt, shame, pain…" have on the experience of healthy adaptive affect [30].

McCullough's group is unique in using the GAF (Global Assessment of Functioning Scale) to assist in determining patient suitability for the treatment.

Ratings of 50 or above on the GAF are deemed to be consistent with suitability for APT. Ratings below 50 indicate a need for more a supportive ego building or defence building intervention. It is felt that the GAF is more useful in assessing suitability than a particular Axis I or Axis II diagnosis.

McCullogh's method makes use of the supportive expressive continuum. Those patients scoring lower on the GAF require more supportive and less exploratory interventions [30]. For patients with scores above 50, expressive techniques can be used to challenge defences and evoke underlying feelings. There is a balance between exploration and support in order to modulate the anxiety level and to maintain and strengthen the therapeutic alliance.

Expressive techniques include confrontation, interpretation, challenging and facilitating the experience of intense affect. Supportive techniques include validation, empathy, reinforcing defences, building social supports, coping skills, advice, reassurance and praise.

A major contribution of McCullough's group is the Achievement of Therapeutic Objectives Scale (ATOS) [32].

The ATOS was designed to assess changes in the key dimensions of psychodynamic psychotherapy: the scale consists of seven dimensions:

- Defence recognition
- Defence relinquishing
- Affect experiencing
- Affect expression
- Level of anxiety, guilt or shame
- Sense of self and degree of self-compassion and self-regard
- Sense of others and degree of relatedness to others

This scale is useful across all forms of dynamic psychotherapy as it is theory neutral. This scale is rated numerically from 1 to 100 with anchor points. The ratings can be made on video and audio recordings or on transcripts of psychotherapy sessions. Ratings are made for each 10-min segment of the session.

For example, a patient who had excellent recognition of maladaptive patterns of thoughts, feelings and behaviours and full awareness of their impacts will be rated at the top end of the scale 91–100. Conversely patients who gains no awareness of the maladaptive patterns even when pointed out by the therapist or disagrees with the therapist's intervention would be rated from 1 to 10.

The ATOS is a very useful contribution to the practice and research of STPPs. It focuses on core components of dynamic psychotherapy. Kristin Osborn and colleagues have produced the ATOS Therapist which can be used to assess therapist competency and adherence to the therapy model [33].

1.6.3 Accelerated Experiential Dynamic Psychotherapy: Diana Fosha

The next quantum leap in the evolution of short-term dynamic psychotherapies was the emergence of Diana Fosha's AEDP (accelerated experiential dynamic psychotherapy). Fosha's work exploded on the psychotherapy scene in North America with the publication in 2000 of her tour de force "The Transforming Power of Affect" [34]. Fosha trained with Davanloo between 1985 and 1988. She later worked with Michael Alpert. Alpert had trained with Davanloo between 1980 and 1983. In the 1990s, he set up an STDP clinic in New Jersey where he worked with Diana Fosha. Alpert called his approach Accelerated Empathic Therapy [35].

Fosha diverged from Davanloo's technique. While retaining the same core dynamic features of the triangle of conflict, she developed interventions to soften and bypass defences. Drawing on and expanding Alpert's work, Fosha formulated an approach to deal with defences in a manner very different to Davanloo. Rather than pressure and challenge the hallmark of Davanloo's interpersonal style, Fosha's method involves "melting" and "bypassing" defences. This is accomplished by maintaining a highly empathic and attuned relational style with patients. The patients' bodily experience of emotion is also elicited which can lead to rapid access to these emotions. The real relationship is acknowledged, and self-disclosure regarding the patient's impact on the therapist is used therapeutically. This entails recognition of the patient's struggles and achievements. These methods are very striking and can lead to rapid "accelerated" progress of therapy.

Fosha stresses that AEDP is healing orientated with the goal of transformation. She refers to "innate, wired-in dispositions for self-healing…" which she has termed "transformance" [34]. A major strategic aim of AEDP is to work with these healthy strivings.

Fosha does not stress explicit emphasis on the transference or use of a specific dynamic focus.

Rather she disconfirms the patient's unconscious negative expectations right from the start of the first session: she welcomes the patient.

By focusing on the development of a secure attachment, there is a reduction in the patient's anxiety which diminishes the need for defensive manoeuvres allowing access to core emotions.

"Moment to moment tracking" is an essential task for the therapist. This requires paying close attention to the patient's experiences as well as the therapist's emotional responses.

An extremely powerful AEDP technique is "metaprocessing". This consists of reflecting on the therapeutic interaction: "What is it like to feel that with me here right now?"

Metaprocessing promotes the development of a coherent autobiographical narrative and a sense of existing in the mind of the other person. For Fosha the unit of therapeutic intervention is not the therapist's comment but the therapist's comment and the patient's response. She is canny in her realization that what is most important is the patient's experience of the therapist's intervention and subsequent response to it.

Fosha has described four psychological states [31]:

State 1: Distress, symptoms, anxiety, shame
State 2: Core emotions
State 3: Transformational affects
State 4: Core state

State 1 consists of the patient presenting in distress with symptoms and dysregulated emotions. Inhibitory emotions such as anxiety, shame and guilt may be evident. Defences are in full force.

Fosha uses therapeutic interventions to help the patient shift into State 2. This involves empathy, attunement and identifying defences. State 2 is the experience of core emotions such as sadness, anger, fear, joy and grief. State 2 is accompanied by feelings of authenticity.

The third stage is facilitated by metaprocessing. Emotions of pride, joy, gratitude and feeling moved may emerge. Conversely feelings of sorrow or mourning what has been lost may arise in response to various reflections.

Fosha calls the deepest level of emotional experience the "core state". This includes feelings of compassion, self-compassion, wisdom and generosity. The patient experiences a sense of calmness, things feel "right" with a coherent self-narrative [31].

Fosha has developed a very well-elaborated theory and methodology, and clearly this brief summary cannot do justice to its complexity and nuances. For further information, the reader can visit the AEDP website for published articles and other resources.

1.6.4 Common Elements of STPPs

It is clear from this brief overview of STPPs that there are many common elements that underpin the workings of psychodynamic psychotherapy. The central and unifying commonality is the recognition of the patient-therapist relationship as the principal therapeutic factor. The incorporation of concepts from attachment theory has enhanced our understanding and our ability to work with this relationship. The process of working with deep emotions is also common across the different forms of STPP.

The recognition of defences and getting past these in order to access emotions are a sine qua non of psychodynamic psychotherapies (Fig. 1.8). Not all of the STPPs make use of a focus, or central theme. This is a prominent feature of those using Luborsky's core conflictual relationship theme and includes Leichsenring and his group in Germany who have published treatment manuals for specific diagnoses [36]. More recently Alessandra Lemma, Mary Target and Peter Fonagy have described the "interpersonal-affective focus" [37].

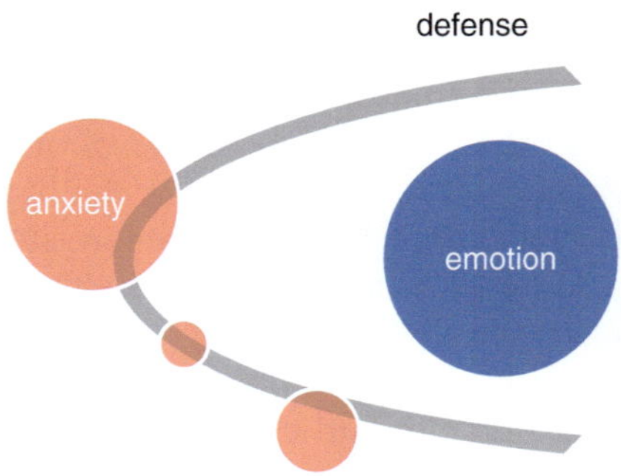

FIGURE 1.8 Anxiety, defence and emotion, the central process in STPP

All of these concepts are similar in identifying recurrent interpersonal patterns as a major focus of psychotherapy. These patterns contain components of the patient's sense of self and his or her feelings towards other people. These patterns are unconsciously repeated and may lead to maladaptive relationships and the emergence of symptoms.

In this manual the term "relational focus" is used for this central thematic idea. In short-term dynamic psychotherapy, a deliberate stance is taken to work with one principal focus. These recurring patterns are linked to the presenting problems and difficulties in the patient's life.

Key Points

- Exploration and expression of deep emotions is a principal change process in all short-term psychodynamic psychotherapies.
- All short-term dynamic therapies aim to access avoided or unconscious emotions that lead to maladaptive patterns of behaviour.
- Getting past defences is a principal strategic aim of these therapies.
- Therapy is facilitated by the development of a strong therapeutic alliance.
- The therapeutic alliance is promoted by the application of findings derived from attachment theory.
- Interpretations are less critical than in classical approaches in contrast to the importance of emotion processing.

References

1. Szekacs-Weisz J, Keve T. Ferenczi and his world: rekindling the spirit of the Budapest school. London: Karnac; 2012.
2. Alexander F, French TM. Psychoanalytic therapy. New York: Ronald Press; 1946. Reprinted by University of Nebraska Press, Lincoln, NE 1980.

3. Palvarini P. Is the concept of corrective emotional experience still topical? Am J Psychother. 2010;64(2):171–94.
4. Balint M, Ornstein P, Balint E. Focal psychotherapy. London: Tavistock Publications; 1972.
5. Gustafson JP. The complex secret of brief psychotherapy in the works of Malan and Balint. In: Gustafson JP, editor. The complex secret of brief psychotherapy. New York: W. W. Norton; 1986. p. 83–128.
6. Malan DH. A study of brief psychotherapy. London: Tavistock Publications; 1963.
7. Malan DH. Beyond interpretation: initial evaluation and technique in short-term dynamic psychotherapy. Part I. Int J Short-Term Psychother. 1986;1:59–82.
8. Malan DH. Beyond interpretation: initial evaluation and technique in short-term dynamic psychotherapy. Part II. Int J Intensive Short-Term Dyn Psychother. 1986;1:83–106.
9. Malan D. The frontier of brief psychotherapy. New York: Plenum; 1976.
10. Balint M. The Doctor, his Patient and the Illness. London: Pitman Med; 1957.
11. Winnicott D. Transitional objects and transitional phenomena. Int J Psychoanal. 1953;34:89–97.
12. Winnicott DW. Ego distortion in terms of true and false self: in the maturational processes and the facilitating environment. London: Hogarth Press and Institute of Psychoanalysis; 1965. p. 140–52.
13. Phillips A. Winnicott. London: Penguin; 2007.
14. Gabbard GO. Psychodynamic psychiatry in clinical practice. Washington: American Psychiatric Press; 1994.
15. Menninger KA. Theory of psychoanalytic technique. New York: Basic Books; 1958.
16. Ezriel H. Notes on Psychoanalytic Group Therapy II: interpretation and research. Psychiatry. 1952;15:119–26.
17. Mann J. Time-limited psychotherapy. Cambridge: Harvard University press; 1973.
18. Bonaparte M. Time and the unconscious. Int J Psychoanal. 1940;427(21).
19. Lindemann E. Symptomatology and management of acute grief. Am J Psychiatr. 1944;101:141–8.
20. Sifneos PE. Short term therapy and emotional crisis. Cambridge, MA: Harvard University Press; 1972. p. 1986.

21. Sifneos PE. Short-term dynamic psychotherapy: evaluation and technique. 2nd ed. New York: Plenum; 1987.
22. Davanloo H. Short-term dynamic psychotherapy. New York: Jason Aronson; 1980.
23. Davanloo H. Basic principles and technique in short-term dynamic psychotherapy. New York: Spectrum Publications; 1978.
24. Luborsky L. Principles of psychoanalytic psychotherapy: a manual for supportive-expressive treatment. New York: Basic Books; 1984.
25. Abbass A, Town J, Ogrodniczuk J. Intensive short-term dynamic psychotherapy trial therapy. Effectiveness and role of "Unlocking the Unconscious". J Nerv Ment Dis. 2017;205(6):453–7.
26. Abbass A. Reaching through resistance: advanced psychotherapy techniques. Kansas City, MO: Seven Leaves; 2015.
27. Abbass A. The emergence of psychodynamic psychotherapy for treatment resistant patients: intensive short- term dynamic psychotherapy. Psychodynamic Psychiat. 2016;44(2):245–80.
28. Abbass A, Town JM. Bona fide psychotherapy models are equally effective for major depressive disorder: future research directions. JAMA Psychiat. 2016;73(9):893–4.
29. Lilliengren P, et al. Intensive Short-Term Dynamic Psychotherapy for generalized anxiety disorder. Clin Psychol Psychotherapy. 2017;24(6):1–9.
30. McCullogh L, Kuhn N, Andrews, et al. Treating affect phobia a manual for short term dynamic psychotherapy. New York: Guilford press; 2003.
31. McCullogh L, Andrews S. Assimilative integration: short-term dynamic psychotherapy for treating affect phobias. Clin Psychol Sci Pract. Spring 2001;8(1):82–97.
32. McCullogh L, Larsen A, Schanche E, Andrews S. Kuhn N. Achievement of Therapeutic Objectives Scale ATOS Scale. 2008. http://www.affectphobiatherapy.com/research-scales/.
33. Osborn K. ATOS therapist 20 point brief rating guides. The Psychotherapy Research Program Harvard Medical School http://www.affectphobiatherapy.com/research-scales/
34. Fosha D. The transforming power of affect: a model for accelerated change. New York: Basic Books; 2000.
35. Alpert MC. Accelerated empathic therapy: a new short-term dynamic psychotherapy. Int J Short-Term Psychother. 1992;7:133–57.

36. Leichsenring F, Schauenburg H. Empirically supported methods of short-term psychodynamic therapy in depression-towards an evidence-based unified protocol. J Affect Disord. 2014;169:128–43.
37. Lemma A, Target M, Fonagy P. Brief dynamic interpersonal therapy. Oxford: Oxford University Press; 2011.

Chapter 2
The Application of Attachment Theory to Short-Term Psychodynamic Psychotherapy

2.1 Child Development

The practice of psychodynamic psychotherapy requires an understanding of child development. Brain development and consequently psychological development are determined by the interaction of genes and the environment [1, 2]. While the growth and development of the brain are genetically programmed, the external environment has a major impact in shaping connections between neural circuits. The infant's actions and the responses from the environment determine which neurocircuits are used frequently leading to the growth and connection of these circuits: "Neurons that fire together wire together". Neural circuits and connections that are not reinforced by activity and experience will be eliminated, a process known as "pruning".

Brain development is subject to critical periods. Genetic programming determines that different neural circuits mature at different time periods. The first 3–6 years of life have an enormous impact. Modifications to brain architecture after these critical periods are much more difficult. Neural circuits responsible for basic sensory and motor functioning mature earlier than those for more complex higher-level functions such as the interpretation of facial expression, language and communication. It is important that the environment responds in an age-appropriate fashion in order that optimal develop-

A. Eppel, *Short-Term Psychodynamic Psychotherapy*, https://doi.org/10.1007/978-3-319-74995-2_2

ment occurs. A deficient or hostile environment can lead to long-lasting alterations in the functioning of the neural circuits. These alterations are much more difficult to change in adulthood. Nevertheless there is some degree of plasticity that can allow for later corrective experiences or intervention.

Childhood development is affected by a range of other factors. Adequate nutrition and housing are paramount. Poverty, war and famine are obviously overriding in their importance. Prenatal nutrition and exposure to toxins or infectious agents can have profound effects. Social and cultural practices and values modify the experience of the growing infant.

Of particular interest to psychodynamic therapists is the relationship between the infant and the mother or other primary attachment figure. The first 3 years of life are particularly important for laying the foundations for a sense of identity and self.

The attachment process and its reciprocal separation and loss are central processes in human life. The attachment system provides physical safety and feelings of security. Proximity to the primary attachment figure regulates the infant's physiological arousal and emotional states. Caregiver response to a distressed infant provides soothing, comfort and reduction in physiological arousal. The secure base provided by the mother gradually allows the infant to explore the world.

2.2 Precursors to Attachment Theory

John Bowlby, a British psychoanalyst, formulated attachment theory beginning in the 1950s. Bowlby worked at the Tavistock Clinic in London, and his theories grew out of the object relations school of psychoanalysis [3, 4, 5]. He strongly disagreed with those analysts such as Melanie Klein who focused exclusively on intrapsychic dynamics and neglected the impact of the external environment.

However other members of the Tavistock Clinic recognized that the relationship between the child and its primary caregiver was vital. In particular one can see precursors to attachment theory in the ideas of Donald Winnicott [6, 7, 8]. Winnicott was a paediatrician who became a pioneering psychoanalyst. He is recognized for his creativity and humility in his dealings with patients. He observed that childhood development depends on the interactions between the infant and the mother. The mother's responses to the newborn infant shape the infant's emotional and psychological development. Infants are unable to fend for themselves. They need to be fed, kept warm and soothed when they feel discomfort or distress. Infants need to be held, touched and spoken to. Based on these responses, the infant develops an inner sense of the external world. Winnicott coined the phrase "the good enough mother" to indicate that the infant's requirements cannot be met 100% of the time and in fact should not be.

Winnicott felt there was an optimal level of maternal responsivity to ensure healthy development and the capacity to become autonomous and confident. Research by Tronick (see below) supports this viewpoint.

With consistent responsiveness by the maternal figure, the infant develops an inner sense that the outside world is benevolent and safe. Over the course of development, he builds up mental representations of himself and of others. In object relations theory, these were referred to as self and object representations. However the fact that the infant's needs are not met 100% of the time means that he has to gradually rely more on his own resources resulting in a modification of his perceptions of external reality. As the child grows, the maternal responsiveness is reduced by small doses allowing the child to develop an increasing sense of independence and self-reliance. Winnicott referred to this as a process of disillusion that fosters the emergence of the infant's "capacity to be alone." The infant has gained some independence from the caregivers and can venture forth in the world.

If the maternal environment is not "good enough," the child will develop some deficits in his self-representation and may view the world as dangerous or hostile. If the external environment is particularly negative, the infant may learn to suppress his true yearnings and urges leading to the development of a “false self” [7]. Winnicott used this concept to describe situations in which the true self is concealed by conforming to external demands at the cost of suppressing inner needs [2–4].

In optimal circumstances, the transition to increasing independence comes in “small and digestible steps”. The infant learns that his own needs may have to be deferred.

Winnicott also conceptualized a transitional zone which bridges subjective experiences and aspects of the external world. Transitional objects such as soft toys stand in place of the primary caregiver. By their association with the mother, they facilitate the development of independence and the capacity to be alone [6].

Winnicott recognized that independence is not an absolute quality rather we all maintain some dependence on others, seeking others and wanting to belong.

2.3 Attachment Theory

Since the time that John Bowlby first conceptualized attachment theory, tens of thousands of articles have been written on the subject and its applications in psychiatry, medicine, child-rearing and psychotherapy [3–5].

It is inspiring to go back to some of Bowlby’s original words because of their clarity and succinctness.

> What for convenience I am terming attachment theory is a way of conceptualizing the propensity of human beings to make strong affectional bonds to particular others and of explaining the many forms of emotional distress and personality disturbance, including anxiety, anger, depression and emotional detachment, to which unwilling separation and loss give rise. [3].

The essence of Bowlby’s theory is that attachment behaviours are genetically programmed.

The infant has an inborn propensity to seek proximity to its mother. Similarly the mother has an inborn biological program of caregiving to respond to the infant’s needs (Table 2.1).

Table 2.1 Key attachment concepts

Proximity seeking	The genetic program that causes infants to seek proximity to their mother or other primary attachment figure
Separation anxiety	The distress experienced by an infant when separated from the primary attachment figure. Indicated by fear, crying and agitation
Secure base	The feeling of safety and security provided by the primary attachment figure that allows them to begin to separate and explore the world
Safe haven	The function provided by the secure base when the infant is in distress and seeks proximity to the attachment figure. Activated by separation, strangeness, pain, hunger, fatigue
Primary attachment figure (PAF)	This is the person who has the most day-to-day interaction with the infant. It may be a parent, a grandparent, a sibling or other caregiver
Internal working models	These are emotional and cognitive representations of the external world. They consist of representations of the self and representations of others. The early attachment relationships form the foundations for emotionally based representations of relationships with others

Proximity seeking is facilitated by the infant's vocalization, smiling, gazing, following and clinging.

These behaviours are evident by 6 or 7 months of age.

The attachment system is an emotional operating system that is comprised of two components: firstly a behavioural or action component and secondly the inner feeling states that trigger and accompany these behaviours. In the infant, the feeling that corresponds to secure attachment is the feeling of being loved. For the mother, the reciprocal inner state is the feeling of loving. Dopamine and oxytocin are two brain chemicals that are intricately involved in the control and experience of attachment and love.

The mother or other primary attachment figures represent a secure base and safe haven. Proximity to the primary attachment figure allays feelings of fear and separation distress.

When the infant is apart from the primary attachment figure, he experiences the feeling of sadness or depression and exhibits behaviours, such as crying, searching and motor agitation.

These behaviours and vocalizations are signals to the PAF and evoke a caring response.

The PAF experiences feelings of concern and the desire to take care of the baby.

If the mother/PAF is unresponsive, the infant experiences too much separation distress and the accompanying affects of sadness, grief or depression. A child in this situation may grow up with a sense of being unloved and unlovable.

Physical and sexual abuses by caregivers are two of the most extreme forms of failed attachment. Abused children grow up with extreme insecurity and mistrust in relationships. Instead of healthy emotion regulation via the attachment dyad, these children experience the terror and extreme psychological pain of abuse. They grow up with the inability to self-soothe and modulate their emotions.

Children with profoundly disturbed attachment relationships develop feelings of intense aloneness. Their adult attachments are insecure and are often characterized by avoidance or anxious preoccupation. As adults they may be diagnosed with complex post-traumatic stress disorder and/or borderline personality disorder.

A child growing up in a nonloving environment may be forced to suppress his true feelings. This often results from the need to accommodate a demanding, abusive parent. The child must suppress his or her authentic emotions and thoughts.

Bowlby described a number of disordered patterns of attachment behaviour. These patterns may develop if the primary attachment figure is unresponsive, rejecting or disparaging to the child's care-eliciting behaviours. Periods of separation from parents, threats by parents/PAFs to withdraw love from the child as a means of discipline and threats by a parent to leave the family have a harmful effect on the development of secure attachment. Bowlby felt that threats bya parent to commit suicide or to kill the other parent were particularly damaging leading to "anxious attachment".

Bowlby described a pattern where a parent induces a premature sense of responsibility in the child. This occurs by making the child feel guilty or by making threats. This in turn can lead to the child developing feelings of anger which he or she cannot express directly. Longings for love and affection may go unfulfilled.

Bowlby described a second pattern of attachment behaviour which he called "compulsive self-reliance" in which the individual attempts to cope with everything by himself. Such individuals block their attachment yearnings and deny any desire for close relationships. They are in fact fearful of developing close relationships or of relying on anyone else in "order to avoid the pain of being rejected" or to avoid the pressure of becoming a caretaker for someone else.

A third pattern described by Bowlby is that of compulsive caregiving. Bowlby postulated that this pattern emerges when the primary attachment parent had some form of incapacity and the only available affectional bond was for the child to take on the behaviour of a caregiver (cf "false self" above).

All of these patterns of anxious attachment are associated with unmet longings for love and feelings of resentment and anger towards those who did not provide it.

2.4 The Mutual Regulation Model: Edward Tronick

Fundamental attachment concepts have received empirical support from the work of Edward Tronick and his research collaborators [10]. Tronick, a developmental and clinical psychologist at the University of Massachusetts in Boston, has made enormous contributions to elaborating the implications of attachment theory for childhood development. Tronick focused on the infant mother dyad. He conceptualized the interaction process between mother and infant as one of emotional regulation. He refers to this as the mutual regulation model (MRM). Tronick's group has identified three types of mother infant interaction:

- Coordinated
- Miscoordinated
- Repair

Coordinated interaction occurs when the mother/PAF is sensitive and attuned to the physical, emotional and communicative needs of the infant. This is evident by the engagement of the mother and baby and by matching behaviour and affect. This is associated with positive emotion in the infant.

Miscoordinated interaction is when there is a lack of attunement or a mismatch between the infant's needs and the response of the primary attachment figure. In this case the infant's needs are not met, resulting in the experience of separation distress, fear, discomfort and inner feelings of badness. If miscoordination is too frequent, the child grows up with insecure attachment and an internal working model of the self of badness and unlovableness that forms a major component of his or her personality. However a certain amount of miscoordination may be required for the infant to be able to differentiate himself as separate from the mother. This is consistent with Winnicott's ideas about "good-enough mothering".

Repair is the movement from a miscoordinated state back to a coordinated state. This may require the mother to engage in soothing and comforting leading to restoration of a mutually resonant interaction, the elimination of disturbing emotions and the return of positive feelings.

The infant's repeated experience of repair leads to a positive inner sense of self, an expectation that things can be repaired. Repair of empathic misattunement facilitates secure attachment. Repair may also promote the acquisition of the capacity to endure deprivation and hardship, that is, the development of psychological resilience.

2.5 Attachment Theory and Psychotherapy

Bowlby initiated the process of applying attachment theory to psychotherapy. Bowlby emphasized that "present modes of perceiving and dealing with emotionally significant persons including the therapist, may be influenced and perhaps seriously distorted by the experiences which he had with his parents during the years of his childhood and adolescence…".

Bowlby's work ultimately led to a true paradigm shift in psychodynamic psychotherapy. Fundamentally his theory is a change of language and concepts that have an analogous relationship to many of the original psychoanalytic ideas (Table 2.2). However because his theories are based on more objective observations, they are more compatible with the sciences of neurobiology and child development.

Bowlby outlined a number of tasks for the therapist:

- To provide the patient with a secure base
- To join with the patient in exploring himself and his relationships

Table 2.2 Comparison of attachment and object relations concepts

Attachment theory	**Object relations**
Secure base	Therapeutic alliance/holding environment
Exploration	Capacity to be alone
Internal working models	Self and object representations
Attunement	Holding environment
Attachment style	Defences
Mentalization existing in the heart and mind of the other	Reflective functioning
Implicit memory	Unconscious
Attachment relationships	Self and objects

- To point out whether the patient's expectations and understanding of the therapist's feelings and behaviours towards him are accurate
- To help the patient see that his relationship patterns and reactions to other people including the therapist may be understood in terms of his early attachment experiences

- Bowlby conceptualized the task of therapy as the need to review with the patient his internal models of attachment figures and of himself. In this way the patient would come to see how these models affected his behaviour and relationships.

Bowlby recognize the importance of non-verbal communication such as tone of voice, stating that this is at least as important as anything the therapist may say. The therapist's respect for his patient is conveyed nonverbally in his attempt to understand the patient's viewpoint.

2.6 Understanding Attachment Terminology and Measures

2.6.1 The Strange Situation

The exploration of the literature on human attachment and its application to psychotherapy is more complicated than it may appear at first sight. Bowlby's original descriptions are characterized by clarity and succinctness the product of a perceptive and reflective intellect.

Numerous methods and instruments have been developed to measure attachment in infants, children, adolescents and adults. These include complex assessment procedures, narrative methods and questionnaires.

The issue of validity is central. Do these instruments all measure the same thing? The answer is clearly no they do not.

The gold standard for the measurement of attachment behaviour in children was developed by Mary Ainsworth [11, 12]. This appears true to the heart of Bowlby's original concepts and observations. However even this methodology has been criticized as being circular.

Ainsworth developed the strange situation procedure. This involves interactions between the mother the infant and a third person. It is applicable to infants between the ages of 12 and 20 months. Each phase lasts 3 min [11].

The parent and infant are brought into a room with a few chairs and some toys on the floor (Table 2.3).

They settle in for 3 min.

A stranger then enters the room. The stranger plays with the infant for 3 min. The parent then leaves the room. This is referred to as the first separation.

After 3 min, the parent returns and the stranger leaves. This is the first reunion.

The parent then leaves the infant alone in the room for the second separation.

After 3 min, the stranger enters the room and stays with the infant.

Three minutes later the parent returns and the stranger leaves. This is the second reunion.

Table 2.3 The strange situation

Action	Subjects in room	Attachment process
Infant and mother enter	Infant and mother	
Stranger enters	Infant, mother, stranger	
Mother leaves	Infant and stranger	First separation
Mother returns; stranger leaves		First reunion
Mother leaves	Infant alone	
Stranger returns	Infant and stranger	
Mother returns; stranger leaves	Infant and mother	Second reunion

Attachment security is defined by Ainsworth "as the state of being secure or untroubled about the availability of the attachment figure" [11, 12].

This paradigm contains the essential components of attachment behaviour: separation from the mother, the secure base and then reuniting with her. Strikingly it is the reunion behaviour that is most critical in illustrating the infant's attachment style.

The attachment classification is based on the infant's reaction to the mother's return.

This is determined by whether the infant seeks proximity and contact with the mother or maintains a distance. Four attachment categories have been derived from the strange situation [11].

Secure Attachment B

The infant is able to explore freely; displays signs of missing the parent particularly during the second separation.

During separation the infant explores less. On reunion the infant greets the parents with a smile, vocalization or gesture. If upset, seeks contact with the parent and when comforted is able to begin exploring again.

Mother is consistently available and responsive to the infant's distress providing a secure base.

Avoidant Attachment A

These infants are able to explore without much need to check on mother.

On separation, the infant exhibits little visible distress when left alone; on reunion, actively avoids the parent, looks away and may focus on toys; if picked up by the parent, may stiffen or lean away and seeks distance from parent.

This pattern is associated with caregivers who are not responsive to the infant's needs or whose response is unpredictable.

Ambivalent or Resistant Attachment C

The infant is distressed on entering the room and displays little exploration.

On separation, the infant is very distressed. On reunion, the infant has difficulty settling and does not find comfort from the parent. He may vacillate between seeking contact and angry rejection with tantrums or inactivity. He is reluctant to leave the mother and start exploring again.

These infants have caregivers that are inconsistent and unpredictable in availability and response.

Disorganized Attachment D

The child's behaviour appears illogical without a goal and exhibits confusion and fear. Behaviour is contradictory with false starts and immobilization. The child appears fearful or apprehensive of the parent and lacks a coherent pattern.

Disorganized attachment is associated with a history of abuse or neglect by the caregiver.

2.6.2 The AAI: The Adult Attachment Interview

The adult attachment interview consists of 20 questions focusing on the individual's relationships with his or her parents during childhood. The patient is asked to describe each parent in turn using five adjectives and then is asked for specific memories illustrating each of these adjectives. The same process can be used for other significant attachment figures [13].

The patient is asked to identify which parent or attachment figure they felt close to as a child and who they would seek help from when they were upset, hurt or ill and to support this with examples.

The interviewee is asked to describe separation experiences from the parents: whether the patient experienced the loss of either parent as a child or as an adult. They are also asked about the current relationship with parents and whether they ever felt rejected or threatened. The interviewees are asked to reflect on how these early experiences may have affected their personality.

The AAI is quite different from the strange situation which is based on observable behaviours. The AAI is a measure of psychological constructs or "states of mind" with respect to the person's attachment experiences [13].

The AAI identifies five categories:

Secure Autonomous F

The subject is able to express a coherent account of attachment experiences. He or she is able to express compassion for his or her parents. The subject can be flexible and display balanced perspectives. He or she is able to appreciate humour.

Dismissing D

These subjects provide an account that lacks coherence. The history is inconsistent or contradictory. They have difficulty with recall. They may display contempt towards particular events or people.

These subjects describe themselves as being strong and independent. They do not identify feelings of needing or depending on others. They minimize negative experiences or present them in positive terms. They are unable to discuss attachment experiences. They are more likely to feel contempt towards attachment figures than sorrow.

Preoccupied E

These subjects have low scores for coherence and high scores for passive or angry preoccupation with their experiences of their parents.

They may provide inaccurate history. They are excessively wordy. Much of what they say may be irrelevant. They are ambivalent and oscillate between blaming and praising the attachment figures.

Unresolved U

These subjects exhibit periods of silence and irrational thoughts. There is a lack of logic in their accounts

Unorganized/Cannot Classify CC

The narrative is incoherent and difficult to follow. The individual may attempt to frighten the interviewer or refuse to speak during the interview [13].

What turned out to be really very dramatic was that parent attachment classification based on the AAI narrative approach was predictive of their children's attachment based on the strange situation methodology [13].

Mary Main realized that the nature of the individual's discourse concerning attachment-related issues was an indication of their own internal working model of attachment.

The adult attachment interview assesses "the patient's state of mind with respect to attachment". Narratives that are accurate, not contradictory, succinct, relevant and clear are indicative of secure attachment states of mind. Conversely an account that lacks coherence and relevance reflects insecure and disorganized attachment states of mind [13].

Individuals who have difficulty being coherent are contradictory. Their responses are brief with little to say about the attachment figures. There may be periods of silence. They cannot recall much about their experiences with key figures. This indicates a dismissing form of insecure attachment.

Individuals who are tangential, are vague and are difficult to follow reflect a preoccupied attachment state mind.

Dissociation and loss of continuity in responses are common in individuals with unresolved or disorganized attachment templates.

It is very important to note that the terminology for different attachment styles and states of mind varies depending on which instruments or paradigms are being employed.

Thus the AAI refers to adult internal working models of attachment, and the nomenclature used is different to that used in Mary Ainsworth's strange situation categories (Table 2.4).

Table 2.4 Comparison of attachment terminology

Adult attachment interview Mary Main	Strange situation Mary Ainsworth
Secure (autonomous) B	Secure
Dismissing	Avoidant
Preoccupied or entangled	Ambivalent
Unresolved/disorganized	Disorganized

Adults with a dismissing attachment template are often clinically categorized as having obsessional, narcissistic or schizoid personality traits. They are fearful of closeness and intimacy and are not in touch with their core emotions. A pattern of devaluation of others and a defensive structure of superiority may be referred to as narcissistic. These patients cannot tolerate genuine intimacy or complements because this risks activating feelings of dependency and vulnerability which was not tolerated by their parents.

Patients who develop a preoccupied state of mind with respect to attachment are "merger hungry" and constantly strive to be in a close relationship. This includes individuals with so-called borderline and histrionic personality types who are very sensitive to separation, loss and abandonment. They display emotional dysregulation and may connect with others via a pattern of helplessness and proximity seeking. Sexuality may be a vehicle to obtain attachment.

Individuals with unresolved/ disorganized attachment models display breakdown in their narrative of experiences of trauma and loss. They are prone to dissociation and projective defences.

One of the effects of psychotherapy may be to create new internal working models that displace some of the older models that arose in childhood. The patient's experience of the nonjudgmental, attuned and securely attached therapist may be a major therapeutic change process.

2.7 Can Attachment Theory Be Applied to Psychotherapy?

Bowlby believed that there was a continuity between infant attachment patterns and adult patterns in close relationships.

This is crucial to the legitimacy of applying attachment theory to psychotherapy.

There are fundamental questions pertaining to whether or not the attachment model is just another metaphor or whether it represents a valid psychobiological process.

The answer to this question is an empirical one. It depends on studies of infants with prospective follow-up as well as studies of adult behaviour. Indeed there is considerable evidence that childhood attachment patterns have a major impact on adult relationships, ability to regulate affect and to maintain positive intimate relationships. There is also considerable empirical literature on the correlation between insecure attachment and the development of psychiatric illness. Adults who are securely attached appear less anxious and more confident in their day-to-day interactions. They are more readily able to express and reflect on their feelings. They exhibit an appropriate balance between autonomy and dependence. They are able to initiate and maintain intimate relationships, to give and accept help and to be trusting of others.

Conversely avoidant or dismissing adults have difficulty with intimacy and openness. They prefer to keep their feelings private and appear socially aloof. They do not like to accept help from others preferring to rely on their own resources. Instead they utilize "deactivating strategies" concealing their inner distress and vulnerabilities by maintaining a composed outward appearance. They are reluctant to accept help or comfort as this may unhinge their inner distress. This may be expressed cognitively in devaluing the ability of others to be helpful and exhibiting a preference for self-sufficiency.

Individuals with preoccupied attachment are very insecure in their intimate relationships, fearful of abandonment and tend to be overly possessive clingy and jealous. They struggle with feelings of rejection and aloneness. They may adopt hyperactivating strategies to maintain proximity in their intimate relationships with intensification of emotional dysregulation [9]. They may attempt to please or placate intimate others at the expense of their own needs and by being self-critical. Their partners may feel pressured and engulfed.

Adults with disorganized attachment may have chaotic relationship patterns and appear disconnected and prone to dissociation. They may exhibit alternating patterns of preoccupied and avoidant attachment. They have difficulty regulating their emotions. They become flooded by overwhelming emotions and under extreme stress may become immobilized.

Is the attachment metaphor superior to the Freudian metaphor? I believe the attachment metaphor is approximates more to scientific evidence. That is because there is a vast research literature on attachment behaviour as well as a solid neuroscientific understanding of this particularly in the work of Panksepp [14].

In this regard adult attachment patterns may be continuous with childhood.

However validity depends on the construct validity of the instruments used to measure attachment. For the adult the gold standard of measurement is the adult attachment interview. Unfortunately this instrument requires extensive training and is also very time-consuming so that the vast majority of studies do not use it. Instead numerous other instruments, frequently self-report questionnaires, have been substituted with attempts to validate them against the AAI. This requires that any review of the attachment literature requires particular attention to the measurement instruments and whether have good correlation with the AAI and have construct validity.

One striking difference between infant attachment and adult attachment is that in adulthood there is more of a symmetrical and reciprocal relationship. In adulthood a sexual relationship is a component of romantic pair bonds.

2.8 Attachment Concepts Used in Psychotherapy

Attachment theory has been applied to short-term psychodynamic psychotherapy in two principal areas. Firstly understanding the patient's psychological development and how early attachment experiences have shaped adult relationship patterns. The concept of internal working models implies that future relationships will be strongly influenced by the experience and internalization of early relationship interactions.

The concepts of secure and insecure attachment are extremely relevant for the conduct of psychotherapy.

Identification of the patient's attachment style is very helpful in understanding his or her views of themselves, of others and relationship patterns.

The second main area of application is in the formation of the therapeutic alliance and the nature of the patient therapist dyad.

Concepts of attunement, responsiveness and provision of a secure base can be applied to the conduct of psychotherapy. The therapist can facilitate optimal emotional regulation within the session by appropriate attunement and responsiveness to the patient's emotional signals. In order to do this, therapist must be attuned on a moment to moment basis to affective changes in the patient [15]. This requires attention to subtle clues and alterations in the patient's facial expression, posture, eye gaze and gesture. Psychotherapy is most effective when there is an optimal level of emotional regulation. Overregulation blocks access to core emotions. Conversely underregulation prevents exploratory work.

The process of rupture and repair which arises out of Tronick's work is extremely relevant to psychotherapy.

As with the primary attachment figure in childhood, the therapist cannot always be in synchrony and attunement with the patient. Inevitable mismatches occur leading to a rupture in the relationship. These ruptures need to be explored and resolved. The repair of ruptures in infancy leads to heightened resiliency. Similarly in psychotherapy the repair of a rupture is extremely therapeutic leading to a corrective emotional experience and greater insight.

2.9 Future Research: The Research Domain Criteria Project

In 2009, the National Institute of Mental Health made a strategic decision to develop new ways of classifying mental disorders based on observable behaviour and neurobiological measures. The goal of this strategy is to improve research in mental illness. NIMH felt that the existing psychiatric classifications have been problematic for research. The new approach taken by NIMH is known as the Research Domain

Criteria (RDoC) project. It provides a new framework for carrying out research based on dimensions rather than categories [16]. This is in contrast to clinical classification systems such as DSM 5 and ICD 11. By "building from the ground up", it is hoped that the RDoC methods will develop classifications that have construct validity.

NIMH has identified five domains in the RDoC matrix: negative valence systems, positive valence systems, cognitive systems, systems for social processes and arousal/regulatory systems. The RDoC construct that is most relevant here is affiliation and attachment.

It is likely that this research will lead to increasing refinement and elaboration of attachment theory and its subcomponents. These concepts will be broken down into more specific dimensions that will facilitate future research.

The concept of attachment embraces selective affiliation to particular individuals. It is determined by activity in neural circuits. It requires the normal functioning of information processing systems to enable social cues and social motivation.

For the normal development of attachment to occur, there needs to be adequate functioning of learning and memory. The infant must be able to recognize facial expressions and other non-verbal signals of emotion in order to form attachments [16].

Future research using these constructs may enhance our understanding of the underlying neurobiology of attachment processes and the effects of disrupted attachment, separation, loss and abuse.

Key Points

- An understanding of childhood development is essential for the practice of short-term psychodynamic psychotherapy.
- Attachment theory provides a framework for understanding the development of relationship patterns.

- Attachment theory explains the development of one's sense of self and identity as well as our expectations and predictions about the behaviour of other people.
- Early attachment relationships have a primary influence on the development of internal working models.
- Internal working models provide a map of the external human environment.
- Internal working models determine our expectations and responses to other people.

References

1. Davies D. Child Development. A Practitioners Guide. 3rd ed. Guilford; 2011.
2. National Scientific Council on the Developing Child. 2007. The Timing and Quality of Early Experiences Combine to Shape Brain Architecture: Working Paper #5. http://www.developingchild.net.
3. Bowlby J. The making and breaking of affectional bonds Brit. J. Psychiat. 1977:130:201–10 and 421–31.
4. Bowlby J. Attachment and loss. Vol. 1: Attachment. 2nd ed. New York: Basic Books; 1982.
5. Bowlby J. Attachment and loss. Vol. 2: Separation: anxiety and anger. New York: Basic Books; 1973.
6. Winnicott D. Transitional objects and transitional phenomena. Int J Psychoanal. 1953;34:89–97.
7. Winnicott DW. Ego distortion in terms of true and false self: in the maturational processes and the facilitating environment. London: Hogarth Press and Institute of Psychoanalysis; 1965. p. 140–52.
8. Phillips A. Winnicott. London: Penguin; 2007.
9. Obegi J, Shaver P, Mikulincer M. A framework for attachment-based psychotherapy with adults. New Therapist. 2009;61:10–21.
10. Tronick E. Dyadically expanded states of consciousness and the process of therapeutic change. Infant Mental Health J. 1998;19:290–9.

11. Ainsworth MDS, Blehar MC, Waters E, Wall S. Patterns of attachment: a psychological study of the strange situation. Hillsdale: Erlbaum; 1978.
12. Solomon J, George C. In: Cassidy J, Shaver P, editors. The measurement of attachment security and related constructs in infancy and early childhood: handbook of attachment. 2nd ed. New York: Guilford Press; 2008. p. 552–98.
13. Hesse E. In: Cassidy J, Shaver P, editors. The adult attachment interview: protocol, method of analysis and empirical atudies in: handbook of attachment. 2nd ed. New York: Guilford Press; 2008. p. 552–98.
14. Panksepp J. Affective neuroscience. New York: Oxford University Press; 1998.
15. Fosha D. The transforming power of affect: a model for accelerated change. Basic Books. 2000.
16. Kozak MJ, Cuthbert BN. The NIMH research domain criteria initiative: background, issues, and pragmatics. Psychophysiology. 2016;53(3):286–97.

Chapter 3
Understanding and Recognizing Emotion

3.1 Background

One of the essential tasks in the practice of psychodynamic psychotherapy is to assist the patient in identifying and expressing deep emotions.

This requires the therapist to have a good understanding of the range of human emotions and to recognize the subtleties of their manifestations.

The emphasis on emotions is one of the principal distinctions in the practice of psychodynamic psychotherapy in contrast to "top-down" cognitive therapies.

The study of emotion is fraught with extraordinary difficulties. To begin with, there are no agreed definitions of the terms "emotion", "feeling" and "affect". The literature can be confusing because the terms affect, feeling and emotion are used differently by different authors.

Terminology varies according to the theoretical framework in which the authors are writing and also in the methodologies used in their research. There are large divergencies between researchers coming from a background in cognitive neuroscience and those working within the framework of affective neuroscience. Methodologies are different.

A. Eppel, *Short-Term Psychodynamic Psychotherapy*,
https://doi.org/10.1007/978-3-319-74995-2_3

Panksepp's work is based on painstaking animal research over several decades [1, 2]. Damasio, a neurologist, studied patients with brain injuries [3, 4]. Functional neuroimaging provides another viewpoint.

While these divisions are artificial, it is nonetheless important to be aware of them in order to understand the literature on emotion.

There is still strong polarization between the cognitive and affective neuroscience views of the nature of emotion. At the basis of this dichotomy is differing views about the relative roles of subcortical and cortical brain systems in the experience and expression of emotion. Cognitive behaviour therapy is based on cognitive neuroscience and learning theory. Psychodynamic psychotherapy emphasizes affective neuroscience, emotions and relational dynamics.

The scientific and intellectual debates have led to multiple research projects including empirical trials of therapy as well as extensive studies of neuroimaging.

These opposing conceptualizations have real-world implications in the application to treatment and treatment outcomes; this in turn has political ramifications in terms of healthcare funding and support.

This division is far from superficial and reflects profoundly different views of the nature of human consciousness and the origins of human emotion.

It is helpful for the psychotherapist to understand the underlying brain mechanisms in the generation of emotions and feelings as this has relevance to the conduct of psychodynamic therapy and the process of change. But first let us look at the clinical aspects of identifying emotions.

3.2 In the Beginning..., Charles Darwin

It was the work of Charles Darwin that established the understanding of the links between body posture, movement and facial expression and the inner experience of emotion [5]. Darwin described the intricate connection between emotion and adaptive action.

Darwin was the first to identify that the expression of emotions was common across most cultures and within the animal kingdom. In his classic work *The Expression of the Emotions in Man and Animals* published in 1872, Darwin described the external manifestations of the emotions, facial expression and bodily movements [5].

The muscles of facial expression are able to convey minute variations associated with specific emotions. Slight changes in the degree of contraction of the facial muscles, subtle alterations in body posture, the pacing of speech, voice characteristics, pitch, amplitude, prosody, variability in laughter, smiling, rapidity of movements and the direction of gaze all help to paint a picture of the underlying emotions.

Darwin identified the following emotions:

- Low spirits, anxiety, grief, dejection and despair
- Joy, high spirits, love, tender feelings and devotion
- Distain, contempt, disgust, guilt and pride
- Surprise, astonishment, fear and horror
- Anger, rage and hatred
- Sadness, grief and melancholy

Smiling occurs across cultures and is evident in newborn infants. About 4–5 months after birth, the human infant is able to discriminate among faces and smile differentially [1].

Smiling involves raising of the upper lip, elevation of the cheeks, brightening and sparkling of the eyes and wrinkling of the lower eyelids (Fig. 3.1).

Guillaume-Benjamin Duchenne distinguished between genuine and false smiles. The genuine smile involves involuntary contraction of the zygomatic muscles elevating the corners of the lips in association with contraction of the orbicularis oculi which causes muscle contraction around the eye and wrinkles at the corners of the eye. The eye opening is narrowed, and the cheeks are raised. The false smile does not include the eye wrinkles and raised cheek. Only truly felt smiles involve the orbicularis oculi. There are also differences in the rate of onset and dissipation of the muscle contractions. A brief upward movement of the eyebrows may also occur in smiling.

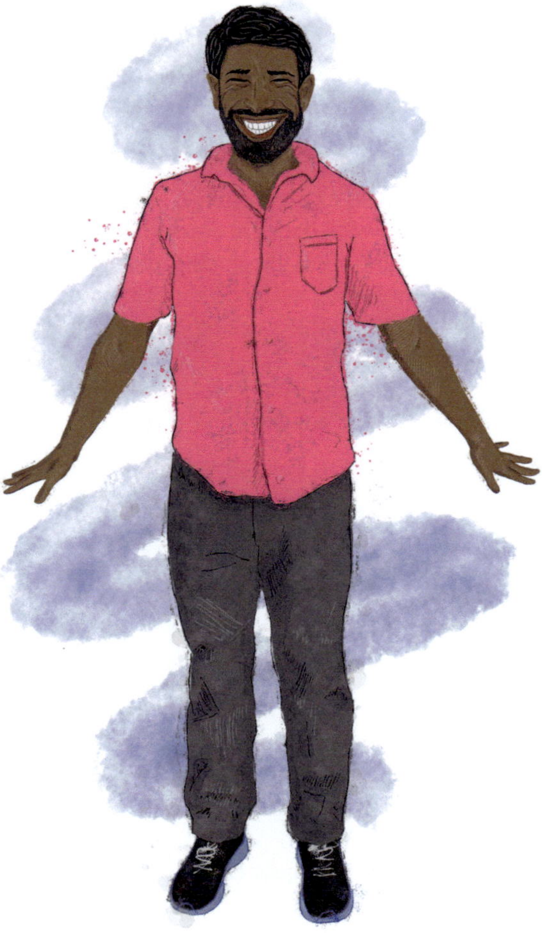

FIGURE 3.1 Joy. (Illustrations by Molly Ferguson www.MollyFergusonArt.com)

The facial expression of sadness involves downward curvature of the corners of the mouth. The inner corners of the eyebrows are drawn up, and the inner corner of the upper eyelid is raised.

Voice characteristics: during mood elevation, there is increase in pitch variability and increased loudness.

During sadness there is decreased frequency level and range of pitch. There is an increased monotone and reduced loudness. In sadness the ends of sentences may drop down to a lower pitch.

Darwin demonstrates exquisite powers of observation of a woman sitting beside him in a train carriage:

> An old lady with a comfortable but absorbed expression sat nearly opposite me in a railway carriage. Whilst I was looking at her, I saw that her depressores anguli oris became very slightly, yet decidedly, contracted but as her countenance remained as placid as ever, I reflected how meaningless was this contraction, and how easily one might be deceived. The thought had hardly occurred to me when I saw that her eyes suddenly became suffused with tears almost to overflowing, and her whole countenance fell. The could now be no doubt that some painful recollection, perhaps that of a long lost child, was passing through her mind. As soon as her sensorium was thus affected, certain nerve cells from long habit instantly transmitted an order to all the respiratory muscles, and to those around the mouth, to prepare for a fit of crying. But the order was countermanded by the will, or rather by a later acquired habit, and all the muscles were obedient, excepting in a slight degree the depressores anguli oris. The mouth is not even opened; the respiration was not hurried and no muscles affected except those which draw down the corners of the mouth [5].

Perhaps no one has more succinctly and evocatively described the complex processes that are the subject of this chapter. Darwin can be an inspiration to psychotherapists learning to identify even the most subtle shifts in facial muscles and tearing of the eyes. Once these glimmers of emotion are observed, it can allow the therapist to facilitate emotional expression. Darwin concludes:

> ...... we can understand how it is, that as soon as some melancholy thought passes through the brain, there occurs a just perceptible drawing down of the corners of the mouth, or slight raising up of the inner ends of the eyebrows, or both movements combined, and immediately afterwards a slight suffusion of tears.

> The expression of low spirits, grief or dejection, due to the contraction of this muscle has been noticed by everyone who has written on the subject. To say that a person is "down in the mouth" is synonymous with saying that he is out of spirits [5].

Darwin's description of rage is equally masterful: he describes changes in circulation and respiration leading to changes in facial colour and distention of veins, heaving of the chest and dilation of the nostrils.

> The body is commonly held erect ready for instant action, but sometimes it is bent forward towards the offending person, with the limbs more or less rigid. The mouth is generally closed with firmness, showing fixed determination, and the teeth are clenched or ground together [5].

Gestures such as raising of the arms or clenching of the fists are common. There may be a glaring of the eyes which are kept open wide (Fig. 3.2). The eyes appear bright. The pupils are contracted. Darwin notes that the retraction of the lips exposing the teeth during rage simulates a threat to bite the offender.

Anger is a less intense form of rage; again the eyes become bright, the respirations increase in rate, the nostrils may widen, the head is erect, the chest wall is expanded, and the feet are planted firmly on the ground (Fig. 3.2). The fists may be clenched. Interestingly the raising of the corner of the mouth on one side exposing the canine tooth is compared by Darwin to that of a snarling dog and may foreshadow aggression. Darwin believes that a sardonic smile is a more attenuated expression of this [5].

I have quoted Darwin at some length to indicate his unique powers of observation and description. Experienced therapists learn to automatically attend to subtle changes in facial expression, voice and posture to help identify and elicit affect. Darwin's work was the first to show the richness and complexity of the expression of emotions. Careful study of his descriptions and the illustrations in this chapter will enhance the readers' powers of detection of emotional signals.

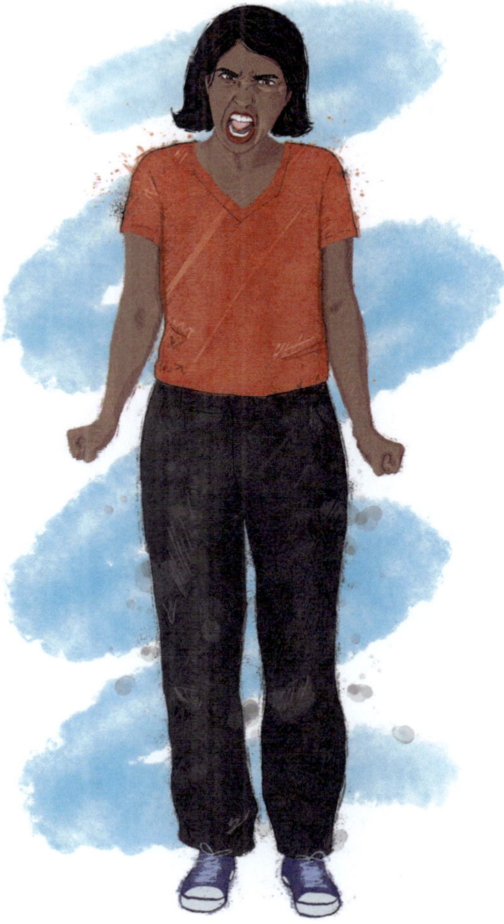

FIGURE 3.2 Anger. (Illustrations by Molly Ferguson www.MollyFergusonArt com)

3.3 The Evolution of Emotion

To understand the psychodynamic model in a more contemporary fashion, we need to draw upon the literature of human and mammalian emotion, neuroimaging and studies of consciousness and self-representation.

These are extremely complex areas. Emotion research has been enhanced by functional MRI and other neuroimaging technologies. However these technologies and paradigms remain limited due to small sample sizes. They are subject to confounding variables and artefacts.

3.3.1 Paul McLean: The Triune Brain

A useful starting point is the framework developed by Paul McLean known as the triune brain [6]. While this is an over-simplification and requires modification, it is nevertheless a model that has great heuristic value. McLean compares the layered nature of the brain to the building of a house where additions are made from the ground floor upwards (Fig. 3.3).

From an evolutionary point of view, the oldest part of our brain is referred to as the "reptilian brain". This evolved hundreds of millions of years ago. Its main function is self-preservation. The reptilian brain controls cardiorespiratory functioning, movement and vision. The reptilian brain is

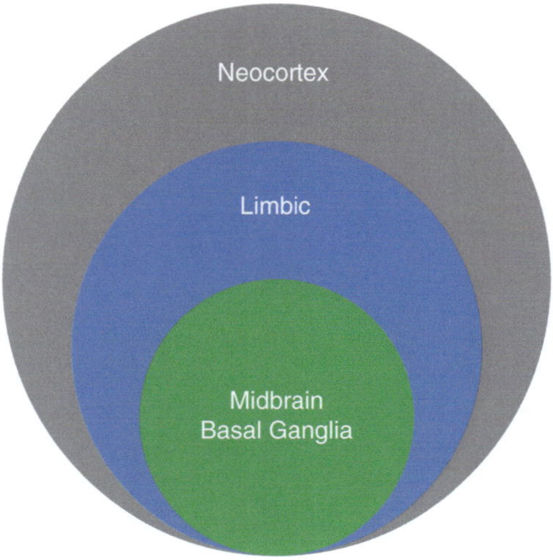

FIGURE 3.3 The triune brain

driven by survival needs. The reptilian brain consists of primitive sensory cortices, the midbrain, the spinal cord, the cerebellum, the upper brainstem, the pons, the thalamus, the reticular system and the basal ganglia.

The reptilian brain is hardwired to produce stereotypical behaviours such as establishing territory and finding a home, hunting, homing, mating, breeding, imprinting, forming social hierarchies and selecting leaders. The establishment of territory is necessary for mating and breeding [p.10]. These are genetically inherited sequential programmed behaviours.

The reptilian brain is the locale of basic instinctual programmes. These are hardwired action processes which contain the machinery for exploration, aggressive dominance displays, sexuality and feeding.

The centre of organization for the reptilian brain is comprised of the basal ganglia. These are located deep in the brain and control the repetitive, stereotyped and ritualized reptilian behaviours. These do not require conscious control. These repetitive behaviours include seeking shelter, seeking food, lying in the sun, courtship and aggressive and submissive displays. [As an aside the repetitive behaviours of obsessive-compulsive disorders may have their origins in these neural circuits.]

The paleomammalian or limbic brain has a cortical layer and overlays the reptilian brain. The word limbic means "forming a border around", and it surrounds the brainstem. The overlay does not replace what is beneath but rather allows exploitation of the reptilian hardwiring and application to additional functions.

The limbic brain comprises a hub for the emotions and neurocircuits related to interpersonal and social behaviours. This includes attachment, separation, maternal caregiving and play.

The limbic system includes the anterior cingulate gyrus, the hippocampus and the amygdala.

The third part of the triune model is the neo-mammalian brain which is coterminous with the neocortex. The neocortex is the site of cognitive and executive functioning. It includes reflection, reasoning, logical thinking, planning, language, symbols and metaphor.

McLean likens the limbic cortex to a primitive television screen giving the mammal a better picture for adapting to its internal and external environment. This appears to be analogous to Damasio's core consciousness. The neocortex can be compared to a much more sophisticated television screen which includes linguistic representations, speech and sound.

McLean [6] states "that the neural machinery does not exist for the reptilian and limbic brains to communicate in verbal terms". With great foresight McLean recognized the implications of this for psychotherapy : verbal insight may be not sufficient for successful treatment.

What is critical is that each of these three domains is superimposed on each other through the course of evolution. The reptilian brain is not replaced by the old mammalian brain which in turn is not made redundant by the neo-mammalian brain. The newer areas of the brain may be able to override the lower levels of function but not replace them.

The link between emotion and action is essential for the survival of the species. The link between fear, changes in facial expression, vocalizations and the action of fight or flight has great survival value. This is both in terms of signalling to conspecifics and parents and preparing the individual to take action in defence or by escape.

3.3.2 The Neurocircuitry of Emotion

Emotional expression involves a sequence of signal, perception, fast appraisal or slow appraisal then action. The hypothesis that there are two routes for processing of emotions referred to as the low road and the high road was popularized by LeDoux [7–10]. The low road mediated at the subcortical level is faster and provides survival value in rapidly responding to external dangers. The high road is slower and is mediated via the cortex and involves cognitive appraisal.

The amygdala has a central function in the emotional neurocircuits. It is connected both to cortical and subcortical areas and plays a special role in the perception of danger and the arousal of fear. The amygdala and its connection to subcortical circuits permit an automatic unconscious response to external threat and the activation of appropriate adaptive actions. External visual, auditory, olfactory or tactile sensory input can activate the amygdala without cortical or conscious processing.

The amygdala is responsible for coding the salience or relevance of incoming stimuli and initiating adaptive action via motor systems to which it is connected.

This may explain human response to nonverbal behaviour occurring outside of awareness. This may have particular relevance to understanding "gut feelings", "love at first sight", empathy, projection and projective identification.

3.3.3 A Dual System for Emotional Processing

Beatrice de Gelder and her group at Maastricht University have proposed a dual system theory of emotional body language with the amygdala as the linchpin of two separate circuits [11, 12].

The role of the amygdala in emotion processes has been known for many decades based initially on lesion studies and in primates involving bilateral ablation of the amygdalae (Fig. 3.4).

(a) A subcortical circuit involves the retina, superior colliculus, pulvinar nucleus of the thalamus, the striatum and amygdala. This mediates the rapid and unconscious perception of emotional body language. This is similar to the nonconscious recognition of faces [7]. This circuit prepares and initiates adaptive behaviour and automatic defensive responses such as withdrawal or freezing. The amygdala assigns valence to incoming stimuli. There is a link to the reward system through the stratum.

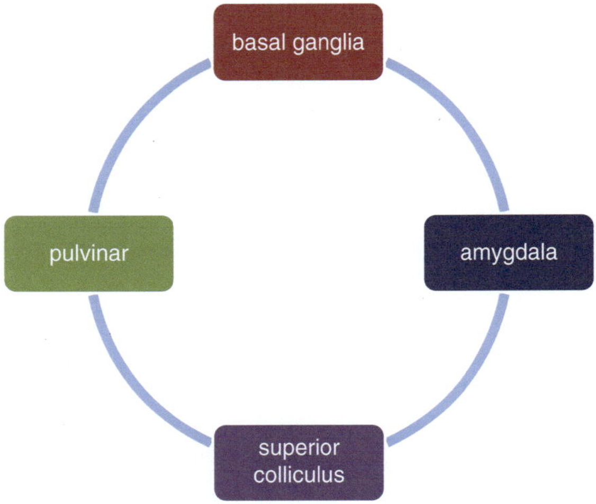

FIGURE 3.4 The Subcortical Circuit

(b)A cortical pathway includes the frontoparietal motor areas and connections between the amygdala, the prefrontal cortex and the ventromedial prefrontal cortex. In this system the incoming stimulus is decoded in the context of past experience and memory. This system analyses at a higher level and computes a decision on a course of action to respond to the stimulus (Fig. 3.5).

These two systems have numerous interconnections. The cortical system involves reflection and decision-making. The meanings of incoming sensory signals need to be interpreted within specific contexts and environments. Also ritualized social gestures and body language may require cognitive interpretation.

There are different terms for describing the subcortical processing of emotional information.

The term "unconscious" is derived from psychodynamics and has theoretical origins. In the research and experimental literature, the term "nonconscious" is used. This is operationally defined as an emotional process in which the subject does not report the presence of a stimulus, and there is evidence that the stimulus has in fact been processed based on changes

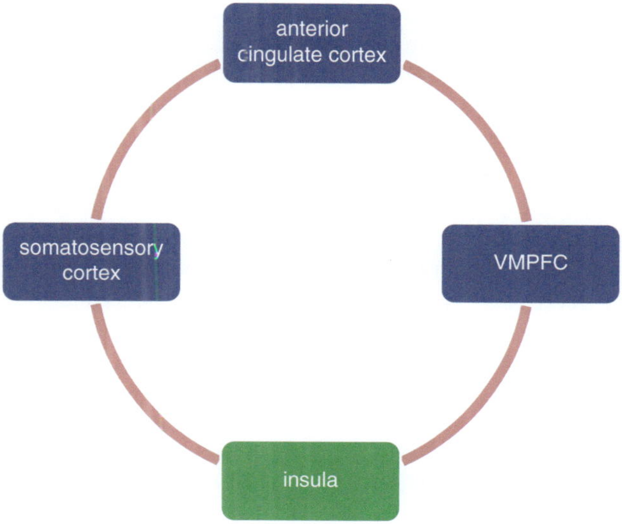

FIGURE 3.5 The Cortical Circuit

in behaviour or physiological measures. The term "automatic" is also used for this subcortical level of processing. Most of the research and observational work has been based on incoming visual stimuli with particular emphasis on facial expressions. However de Gelder and colleagues have demonstrated that other emotional stimuli follow the same root and include body posture. Nonconscious processing of emotional stimuli is accompanied by physiological changes in heart rate, pupillary dilation and rate of eye blinking. There are also changes in facial expression that may be picked up by observers.

Interestingly automatic nonconscious changes in facial expression are mediated by the basal ganglia. Intentional changes to facial expression are controlled by the cortex via the pyramidal motor system. This may explain the difference between genuine and nongenuine smiles as described by Duchenne.

Although this has been described as a dual processing system in actual fact, there are many feedback loops between the subcortical and cortical centres involved in these neurocircuits. The two systems modulate each other. The cortical level may inhibit activity in the subcortical areas. Conversely subcortical areas may activate the orbitofrontal cortex and anterior cingulate cortex.

The dual system of emotional processing has great relevance to the practice of psychodynamic psychotherapy. Key processes in therapy involve eliciting core emotions which have their origins in the subcortical neurocircuits. These emotions need to be processed then to be reflected upon and related to past memories and current context. This is referred to as meta-therapeutic processing and is one of the key change factors in psychodynamic psychotherapy.

3.4 Damasio Where Do I Feel Emotion?

Over several decades Antonio Damasio, a neurologist and brain researcher at the University of Southern California, has made a major contribution to understanding the neurobiological basis of emotions [3, 4]. A major thesis of Damasio's theory is that "feelings" are mental experiences of bodily states. He famously coined the phrase "Descartes' Error". In his book of the same name, he argues that Descartes' felicitous mantra "Cogito ergo sum" was completely wrong [13]. Descartes' mistake was to insist on a separation between the body and the mind. Damasio's views are the exact opposite: that the experience of affect and of consciousness are firmly rooted in the body. Damasio distinguishes "having a feeling" from "knowing the feeling" and from reflecting on feeling. Bodily state changes are topographically mapped onto the upper brainstem and cerebral cortex. Changes in these neural maps initiate action programmes, corrective responses to the deviations from the body baseline. Examples of action programmes include fight and flight and freezing in the face of aggressive threats [4].

Emotional stimuli may come from the outside world in the form of threats leading to fear. They can also come from internal changes. The brain can activate the emotional body state representations even in the absence of specific external or internal triggers.This can be done through, for example, imagination. This implies that there is some form of central representation of bodily changes.

This point is very important for psychotherapists in that it allows us to understand the emotions of others as well as predict our own future emotional response by means of simulating these emotions within ourselves. This also may be the basis for empathy. (See Chap. 5 of this volume.)

Damasio has also proposed that each basic emotion category is correlated with a distinct body state. This refers to the "felt changes" associated with different emotions. For example, happiness is associated with increased sensation in the whole body, whereas anger involves increased sensation in the arms, head and torso. Sadness is associated with decreased feeling in the arms and legs and increased feelings in the chest. Disgust is accompanied by increased sensation in the throat and digestive track. This supports the idea that emotions do have distinct physiological and felt bodily patterns.

The source for the sensation of bodily changes comes from interoceptive signals from the viscera, skeletal muscles and the internal milieu [3]. The interoceptive system consists of neural pathways and nuclei that detect and map signals from the body and internal organs. This includes perception of pain, temperature, proprioception and vestibular sensations.

The vagus nerve conducts signals from the cardiovascular, respiratory, gastrointestinal and genitourinary systems to the lower brainstem.

All this information is collected in the upper brainstem in an area known as the periaqueductal grey (PAG) which may be the locus for the formation of whole body maps of body states and provides the basis for the emergence of feeling states [4]. Neuroimaging studies have suggested that the insula has an important role in mediating interoceptive inputs and the generation of feelings.

3.4.1 The Insula

Craig [14] writes that the insula contains a neural representation of the state of our body and is a substrate of how we feel. The insula is an interoceptive cortex that receives inputs from the viscera, proprioception, vestibular sense, pain and temperature.

The insula is connected to the anterior cingulate cortex and regions of the prefrontal cortex. The insula may provide a continuously updated representation of the current state of our body and how we feel [11].

3.5 Why Are Emotions Contagious?

Another quality of emotions is that they are contagious. This may have a role in regulating social behaviour. The process of empathy allows us to know how another person is feeling. It may be a form of internal simulation. This may account for the so-called mirror phenomena whereby our own feelings are activated when observing the experience of another person. For example, another person experiencing anger or disgust may lead to our own feelings of anger or disgust. The experience of empathic emotional contagion depends on the closeness of the relationship to the person being observed.

3.6 Paul Ekman

Ekman surveyed emotion researchers and asked which emotions they felt were empirically validated out of the following choices:

Fear, anger, awe, compassion, contempt, disgust and embarrassment
Envy, gratitude, guilt, shame, pride and hatred
Happiness, love and surprise

There was a general agreement among the researches that the following five emotions have been empirically established [15]:

Table 3.1 Core and Social Emotions

First order	Second order
Anger, rage	Envy, jealousy
Fear	Guilt, shame
Sadness	Jealousy
Happiness, joy	Pride
Disgust	Contempt

Anger, fear, disgust, sadness and happiness (Table 3.1).

3.6.1 Higher-Order Social Emotions

These emotions are complex and have meaning only in a social context. They are cognitively experienced and require rational thought, evaluation and deliberation. These emotions may serve a social rather than an interpersonal function. For example, shaming is a method of social control that may be exercised in the interests of the social group superseding those of the individual. Similarly guilt ensures conformance to socially demanded behaviours.

- Pride
- Shame and embarrassment
- Guilt
- Jealousy
- Envy

The experience of jealousy requires a higher cortical reasoning capacity, the ability to appreciate the intentions and emotional experience of others [cf. mentalization].

3.7 Jaak Panksepp

Panksepp was the most prominent pioneer in the study of animal and human emotions. He identified the critical importance of genetically hardwired subcortical affective systems.

He coined the term "affective neuroscience". He was critical of Ledoux's early work for not recognizing the importance of the subcortical basis of emotions. He also did not agree with Damasio's conceptualizations. Damasio, who had written the book *Descartes' Error* [13], led Panksepp to refer to "Damasio's Error". In contrast to Descartes' "I think therefore I am", Panksepp suggested that "I feel therefore I am" may be closer to the truth [1].

Jaak Panksepp conducted animal research over many decades and elucidated seven basic emotional systems that are common to all mammals. He referred to these as the "blue ribbon, grade A" emotional systems [1]. Panksepp identified neural circuits that are the basis for these emotional systems. He believed that these seven emotional systems are genetically programmed. In addition he identified key neurotransmitters connected to the circuits. He used capitalization to distinguish the circuits from the everyday use of these words and originally named them as follows: SEEKING, RAGE, FEAR, LUST, PANIC, CARE and PLAY.

According to Panksepp, the basic emotional systems are located in the subcortical areas of the brain. Damage or removal of the cortex does not interfere with the circuits. Such animals continued to exhibit seeking behaviours, fear, anger, sexuality, maternal care and playfulness.

The emotional systems are activated by internal and external stimulations that are related to survival. The emotional systems are experienced as visceral affect and are linked to specific action patterns.

During the course of infant development, cognitive representations of the primary emotions develop in the neocortex. An analogy may be a television set where information is activated along various electrical and radio circuits that at a higher level are translated into coherent images.

3.7.1 The Seeking System

The seeking system is a motivational system that instigates exploration and anticipates excitement. This system programmes interest in the external world and exploration.

This exploration is critical to human development and the learning process. The seeking system is essential to survival. Exploration of the environment permits the discovery of food and shelter. At the secondary level, this involves curiosity and motivates the individual to search for things that they need or desire. It is the basis for human curiosity. Underactivity of this system is associated with depression; overactivity of the system may be the basis for manic-type behaviours. The seeking system is necessary for animals to acquire the needed resources for survival. The seeking system allows the animal to find and store food. It is associated with the ventral tegmental area and nucleus accumbens. It is related but not identical to the more widely used concept of the reward system.

The seeking system is directed towards environmental rewards and associated with addictive seeking behaviours and dopamine neurotransmission.

3.7.2 The Rage/Anger System

Rage and anger develop when the animals' actions are blocked. This system is essential for survival and is required for defence against predators and rivals (Fig. 3.2).

3.7.3 The Fear System

This system is activated by danger and threat. This circuit is associated with fight, flight and freezing. Maladaptive functioning of the system may be the basis for clinical anxiety disorders (Fig. 3.6).

3.7.4 Separation Distress and Social Bonding Systems

These are the circuits that underlie the inborn programmes for attachment behaviour: proximity-seeking and separation distress (Fig. 3.7). There is a reciprocal circuit in the mother which activates responsivity to the infant with caring behav-

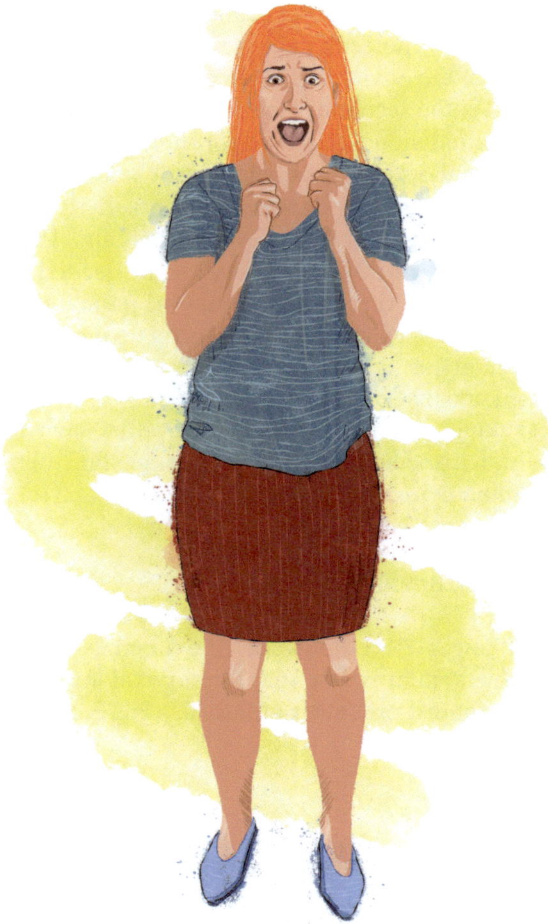

FIGURE. 3.6 Fear. (Illustrations by Molly Ferguson www.MollyFergusonArt.com)

iours. The second-order representation of this circuit includes feelings of affiliation and love.

Panksepp discovered that opioids relieved separation distress in animals. This may be the link between problems of opioid addiction and individuals with severe disorders of attachment. Oxytocin also alleviates separation distress.

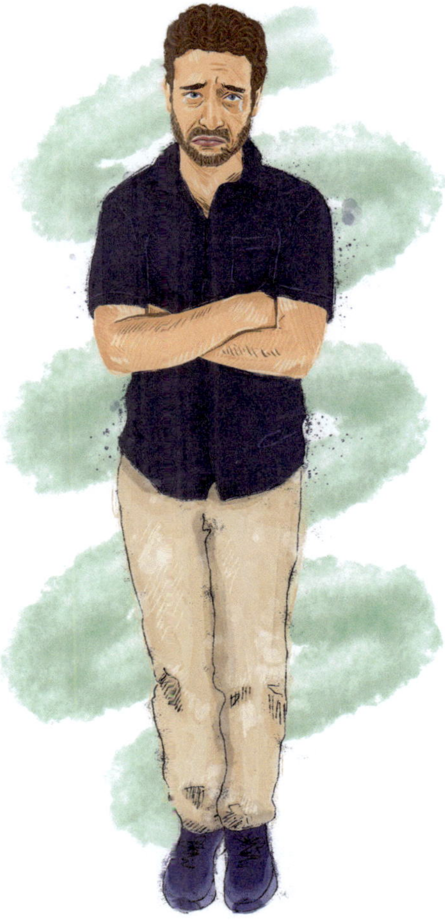

FIGURE 3.7 Sadness. (Illustrations by Molly Ferguson www.MollyFergusonArt.com)

3.75 Sexual/Lust

The neural circuits involved in sexuality are influenced by a number of hormones and neuropeptides. This includes oxytocin, endorphins, prolactin and vasopressin.

3.7.6 Joy/Rough-and-Tumble Play

This neural circuit promotes social engagement and interactions that we refer to as play. These behaviours lead to feelings of joy and exhilaration. Playfulness is essential for early psychological and social development.

Panksepp conceptualized reciprocal interactions between the subcortical and cortical regions in the expression and regulation of emotions. When emotions are generated in the subcortical neural circuits, they may lead to activation of the cortical centres. He agrees that the cortical regions are involved in appraisals of emotion which involve perception, attention and memory retrieval; cortical regions can suppress or "turn off" the subcortical emotional responses. These connections however are bidirectional so that cortical regions may activate the subcortical emotional systems. In other words emotional expression and experience entails both top-down and bottom-up interactions.

3.8 Conclusions: Why Does This Matter?

This model has some explanatory relevance to methods used in psychotherapy. Psychotherapy involves the facilitation of new conscious emotional experiences while old memories are reactivated. Memories are then reconsolidated within the hippocampal cortex.

Conscious experience of unconscious emotions seems to be required in psychotherapy. Representations are made available to working memory which is necessary for long-term memory consolidation [16].

In simple terms, the debate between affective neuroscience and cognitive neuroscience revolves around the relative importance of subcortical emotional forces in contrast to emotion modulation that is based on cortical processes (Fig. 3.8).

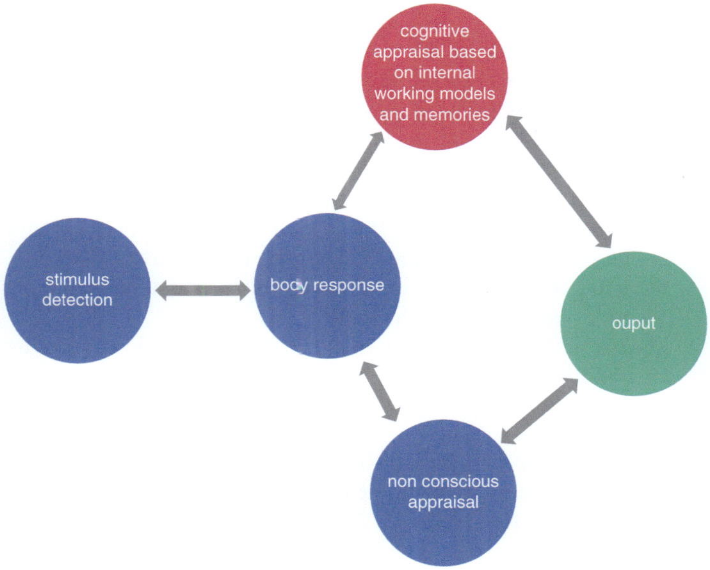

FIGURE. 3.8 Dual Processing of Emotion

Key Points

- There is agreement among researchers that several key emotions are universal.
- The ability to recognize emotional cues is essential for psychodynamic psychotherapists.
- The dual processing theory of emotion is applicable to psychodynamic psychotherapy and explains the working through of emotions and the therapeutic effect of reconsolidation of memories.
- Emotions are conveyed by verbal and non-verbal communication.
- Emotions are experienced viscerally, psychologically and bodily.

References

1. Panksepp J. Affective neuroscience. Oxford; 1998.
2. Panksepp J. Textbook of biological psychiatry. Hoboken: Wiley-Liss; 2004.
3. Damasio A. The feeling of what happens: body and emotion in the making of consciousness. Orlando: Harcourt; 1999.
4. Damasio A, Carvalho G. The nature of feelings: evolutionary and neurobiological origins. Nat Rev Neurosci. 2013;14:143–52.
5. Darwin CR. The expression of the emotions in man and animals. 1st ed. London: John Murray; 1872.
6. Maclean P. A triune concept of the brain and behaviour. Toronto: University of Toronto Press; 1973.
7. LeDoux JE. Emotion circuits in the brain. Annu Rev Neurosci. 2000;23:155–84.
8. Pessoa L, Adolphs R. Emotion processing and the amygdala: from a "low road" to "many roads" of evaluating biological significance. Nat Rev Neurosci. 2010;11:773–82.
9. Adolphs R. Emotion. Curr Biol. 2010;20(13):R549–52.
10. Adolphs R. The biology of fear. Curr Biol. 2013;23:R79–93.
11. de Gelder B. Towards the neurobiology of emotional body language. Nat Rev Neurosci. 2006;7:242–9.
12. Tamietto M, de Gelder B. Neural bases of the non-conscious perception of emotional signals. Nat Rev Neurosci. 2010;11(10):697–709.
13. Damasio A. Descartes' error: emotion, reason, and the human brain. New York: Penguin; 2005.
14. Craig AD. How do you feel? Interoception: the sense of the physiological condition of the body. Nat Rev Neurosci. 2002;3(8):655–66.
15. Ekman P. What scientists who study emotion agree about. Perspect Psychol Sci. 2016;11:31–340.
16. Smith R, Lane RD. The neural basis of one's own conscious and unconscious emotional states. Neurosci Biobehav Rev. 2015;57:1–29.

Chapter 4
A Critical Review of Psychotherapy Research

4.1 Background

Evidence-based medicine has had a profound effect on research in the health sciences. Over the course of three decades, the standards for conducting and evaluating research have undergone a major transformation. The double-blind randomized controlled trial has been established as the "gold standard" for determining treatment outcomes [1–3].

Evidence-based medicine has been adopted internationally and has given rise to parallel paradigms in psychology and related disciplines. The American Psychological Association adopted the term "evidence-based practice in psychology" which requires similar standards of evidence [4].

The widespread adoption of evidence-based principles has resulted in researchers and clinicians becoming much more critical and sceptical in their thinking. Students in the health sciences are now required to develop critical appraisal skills in order to determine the validity and applicability of research studies. Clinicians are better able to identify methodological shortcomings of studies and to adopt a more sceptical attitude to published research. This is a healthy change. Conversely the quality of published research has come under scrutiny. So much is this the case that several leading scholars claim that the majority of published medical research is methodologically flawed and even false [5]. This is quite an

A. Eppel, *Short-Term Psychodynamic Psychotherapy*,
https://doi.org/10.1007/978-3-319-74995-2_4

astonishing claim from such eminent authorities. These concerns can lead to a nihilistic attitude to research endeavours. It is therefore essential for psychodynamic psychotherapists to understand the scientific literature in order to evaluate which treatments work for which problems.

4.2 History

Historically psychodynamic psychotherapy has faced long-standing criticism about its effectiveness. Since its inception the scientific legitimacy of psychoanalysis has been questioned. Many distinguished philosophers of the scientific method including Karl Popper believed that psychoanalysis was a "pseudoscience" [6].

Freud's original goal had been to develop a scientifically based model of the human brain. This was not possible due to the limited understanding of neurophysiology and neuroscience at the time. As an alternative he devised a theory of psychological functioning based on meticulous observation of individual patients. Freud's conceptual model was based on analogies and metaphors. Concepts such as the ego, the id and the superego are not entities in themselves and do not correspond to any neuroanatomical or neurophysiological structures. They are conceptual proxies. The language of psychoanalysis was of necessity essentially metaphorical but nevertheless has had enormous influence in understanding psychological processes.

Central to the critique of psychoanalysis was that none of its tenets could be subject to refutation a sine qua non of the scientific method formulated by Karl Popper [6].

Pseudosciences have been characterized by Lilienfeld as lacking methodological safeguards against confirmation bias [7]. Confirmation bias is the tendency to seek out evidence consistent with the practitioner's hypotheses and to dismiss evidence that does not support his theory.

Karl Popper's criticisms of psychoanalysis as practised in the last century have validity. However over the past three decades, the study of psychodynamic psychotherapy has made substantial progress, and it has been possible to formulate hypotheses and predictions that are subject to falsifiability and refutation. Many prospective studies have been done to determine the impact of childhood events on the future development of personality and behaviour. This has provided more valid information in contrast to psychoanalysis which relied on retrospective study based on patients' reports. The impact of therapeutic methods has been studied in dozens of randomized controlled trials, and it has also been possible to study specific components of psychodynamic therapy and formulate refutable hypotheses.

Cognitive behavioural therapy has been the most extensively researched psychotherapy. Randomized controlled trials have been carried out for the treatment of depression, anxiety disorders, post-traumatic stress disorder, eating disorders, pain, insomnia, substance use, schizophrenia and physical symptoms. There have been far fewer randomized controlled trials in psychodynamic psychotherapy. However, over the past three decades, there has been a growth in high-quality research of psychodynamic psychotherapy. Active research groups exist in the United States, Canada, Germany, the Netherlands, Sweden, Denmark and the United Kingdom.

4.3 Basic Principles of Psychotherapy Research: Effect Sizes

The basic principles of outcome research involve testing one treatment against a proven active treatment and a placebo. Samples are drawn from a defined population. Measures of outcome are evaluated according to significance and effect size (Fig. 4.1). Effect sizes are the most important measures in

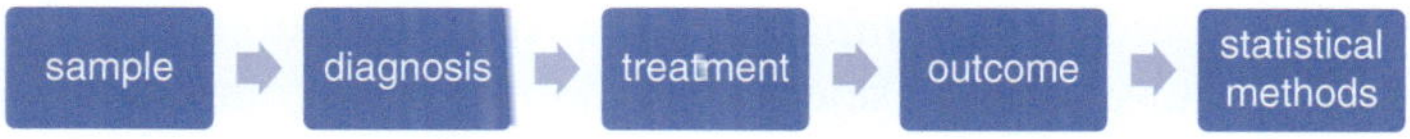

FIGURE 4.1 The research process

studies of psychotherapy and other treatments. To demonstrate that the therapy is effective, it must have an effect size greater than zero. The effect size must be large enough to be clinically relevant. For example, consider a study comparing the outcomes in the treatment of depression using a specific form of psychotherapy and an inactive control. A valid measure of outcomes is essential, and in this hypothetical example, let us say that the Beck Depression Inventory (BDI) was used. In the active psychotherapy group, the average (mean) reduction in BDI scores was 8 points. In the inactive group, the reduction was 5 points. These results were found to be significant, meaning that the results were unlikely to have been produced by chance. The question of interest however is whether the difference in effect sizes is clinically relevant. Does a difference of 3 points on the BDI support the use of the active treatment?

To answer this question we need a standardized statistical measure of effect size. There are several such measures, but Cohen's d is one of the most frequently cited in psychotherapy studies. Cohen's d is calculated from the mean differences of an effect. An effect size is considered small if $d = 0.2$, medium if $d = 0.5$ and large if $d = 0.8$ or higher. However these values must be related to the clinical impact. Small effect sizes can be associated with important clinical benefits.

4.3.1 *Bias*

Research methodology is predicated on the attempt to eliminate bias and false conclusions.

Bias is a systematic error leading to erroneous results. Bias may lead to false-positive or false-negative results. Bias can occur at any phase of a study.

Selection bias refers to differences between the populations that are to be compared. To prevent this, subjects in all study groups must be selected randomly. There must not be any selection of subjects that are more likely to respond to one treatment or another. Subjects must be allocated to the treatment groups in a random fashion. Random allocations are made in sequence and must be hidden from those making the allocations. This is known as random sequence generation.

If subjects or therapists are aware of the treatment, this may bias the responses to interventions or rating of treatment outcomes. Therefore raters of outcomes must be "blinded" as to which treatment the subject received.

Allegiance bias may occur when the researchers have a particular allegiance to one method of psychotherapy leading to unconscious bias. This can be assessed by measuring the correlation between therapist allegiance and outcome measures.

Publication bias refers to the higher likelihood that studies with beneficial outcomes will be published in journals. Research with positive results are more likely to be submitted for publication and more likely to be published. This is why all clinical trials need to be registered prior to initiation. That way the results of nonpublished trials can be used in analyses. Publication bias can be assessed by a number of methods. One of these methods is known as a "funnel plot." This involves plotting effect sizes against sample sizes. If the resulting graph is shaped like a funnel, it indicates that there is no publication bias.

Reporting bias refers to investigators publishing only those outcomes that are significant.

Bias may also result from participants dropping out of studies and being lost to follow-up.

This results in incomplete outcome data. The impact of dropping out must be included in any analysis using "intent-to-treat" analysis. Studies must be of adequate duration with follow-up to determine if treatment effects are maintained.

Sample sizes must be large enough to avoid results that may occur by random chance alone. Comparison groups must be similar.

In medication trials those administering the treatments are blinded to active treatment versus placebo. Placebos are made to look identical to the comparator active drug. In the case of psychotherapy research it is not possible for the therapist or the patient to be blind to the treatment method. Psychotherapy is not unique in this. There are similar difficulties in carrying out surgical research. It has been estimated that 40–50% of surgical patients are receiving treatment that is not evidence-based [8].

4.4 Research Methodologies

The randomized controlled trial is considered the highest standard of evidence in medical science. A hierarchy of evidence has been outlined by Haynes et al. in their work on evidence-based medicine [1]. The American Psychological Association identified empirically supported psychological treatments to demonstrate equal effectiveness to biological treatments [4]. Empirically supported psychological treatments generally require a manualized approach that has been studied in randomized controlled trials for specific diagnostic indications.

A second research methodology involves the analysis of process measures in relation to outcomes [9–21]. This type of research is greatly facilitated by video recordings of individual sessions and analysis of detailed segments. Leigh McCullough and the Harvard group established a 10-year programme of this type of research which is being continued by her associates following her untimely death [22]. This approach has trans-theoretical application by identifying the relational mechanisms of change (Chap. 1). Different schools of therapy may utilize different concepts and terminology which may in fact have an underlying common basis or mechanism.

Evidence-based medicine pioneered at McMaster University in Hamilton Ontario advocates the identification of the best available evidence to bring to bear within the clinical encounter. The best available evidence is combined with the patient's particular needs and preferences.

Evidence-based approaches are not universally accepted as applicable to psychotherapy or even to psychiatry. Gupta [23] has been an outspoken critic of EBM based on its underlying epistemological assumptions. She questions the implicit values and premises of evidence-based medicine and whether it can be ethically applied to psychiatry.

Choice of measures is often determined by the theoretical framework of the therapeutic method. The most straightforward measures are established and validated measures of symptom improvement such as depression or anxiety rating scales. However the therapy may not be directed solely to symptom change. In the case of cognitive behaviour therapy for depression and anxiety, outcome measures are quite straightforward and include such well-established instruments as the Beck Depression Inventory, the DASS and GAD 7. In psychodynamic therapy, outcomes are broader and include improvement in self-image and self-perception, improvements in relationships with others, relinquishing of maladaptive interpersonal patterns and improved access to emotions. Measurement of these changes can be difficult.

4.4.1 Randomized Controlled Trials and Meta-Analyses

To overcome the problem of small samples, the method of meta-analysis is used.

This is a statistical procedure in which the results of multiple studies are combined in order to yield an adequate sample size.

In order for a meta-analysis to be valid, it is important that each of the individual studies is measuring the same thing in similar populations. This means that diagnostic assessments and treatment outcomes must meet the same standards and that measures are the same or at least compatible. This follows the well-known maxim "garbage in leads to garbage out".

The results of a meta-analysis can only be as good as the studies on which it is based.

In studies of psychiatric disorders, it can be difficult to ensure that diagnostic groups are equivalent. This is an intrinsic problem within psychiatry and psychology because of the still rudimentary nature of the classification of mental illness. Criteria for many different diagnoses overlap. As a result patients are often diagnosed with multiple "co-morbid" disorders. This comorbidity is in part an artefact of our classification systems and has led the National Institute of Mental Health to develop an alternative approach using dimensions: the Research Domain Criteria Project [24].

Heterogeneity refers to the case when there are differences between the studies included in a meta-analysis. Studies may differ in the type of patients included, the type of interventions and the measures of outcome. There may also be statistical and methodological differences. If differences are found between studies, the results of the meta-analysis may not be valid. Studies cannot be pooled. Statistical tests are available to measure the degree of heterogeneity.

Meta-analyses can be performed with the assumption that all the studies are sufficiently similar with similar effects. This is referred to as "the fixed effects model". When it is assumed that the effect is not the same in all studies, a different statistical procedure is used known as "the random effects model". The fixed effects model is more powerful. When a fixed effects model is used even though heterogeneity exists, the combined pooled estimate of results may give too much weight to larger studies. The choice of using a fixed or random effects model can have a major impact on the pooled results.

The results of a meta-analysis are graphically portrayed in a "forest plot" also known as a "blobbogram". The studies included in the meta-analysis are listed showing effect sizes with point estimates and confidence intervals. The pooled results are displayed at the bottom of the plot.

In the centre of the plot is the "vertical line of no effect". If the results cross this line, it means there is no effect of the intervention.

4.5 Critical Reviews: The Current State of Research

A major overview of research in psychotherapy was undertaken by Dragioti et al. [25]. This contained 173 individual studies and 247 meta-analyses. Treatments included CBT, psychodynamics, family systems therapy, cognitive remediation, dialectical behaviour therapy, IPT, mindfulness, problem-solving therapy, acceptance and commitment therapy, supportive therapy and counselling. A lesser number of studies of behavioural activation, behaviour modification, EMDR, motivational interviewing, prolonged exposure and trauma-focused therapy were included.

Of these published results, 196 showed significant benefits of the psychotherapy. The authors however felt that only 16 meta-analyses, that is, 7% provided "convincing" evidence of psychotherapy effectiveness. Six of these studies were of CBT and one of meditation therapy.

The authors felt that there was a large degree of heterogeneity in 130 of the meta-analyses. The impact of small-study effects and overrepresentation of studies with positive significant findings brought into question the conclusions of these studies. They found problems with systematic biases including bias related to the researchers' allegiance to a particular school of therapy. They ascertained that allegiance bias could inflate treatment effects by almost 30%. Publication bias was also deemed to overestimate effect sizes. These authors pinpointed problems with inadequate randomization, small sample sizes and incomplete reporting. Dragioti et al. chose a threshold of 1000 participants as an adequate sample size. Only 16 meta-analyses out of 247 met this threshold and met the standards for "convincing evidence". Of these, five involved CBT; seven involved "mixed" psychotherapy. Very few psychodynamic psychotherapies were included in the 247 meta-analyses.

Jan Scott in an editorial in the same issue of the journal described research in psychotherapy as "imperfect and still evolving" [26]. Factors that are difficult to define in meta-analyses are the skill level of the therapists and the fidelity to the therapy model. Scott calls attention to the need to monitor potential harms as well as benefits when evaluating psychotherapy outcomes and the need to conduct more studies to determine which specific therapies work for which types of patients.

Dragioti's study had some limitations of its own. Only randomized controlled trials that were contained in meta-analyses were included resulting in 173 eligible RCTs. This methodology may have excluded relevant randomized controlled trials that were not part of any of the meta-analyses studied.

They also excluded meta-analysis that contained less than ten individual trials and may have missed meta-analyses with large total sample sizes though with less individual studies.

Contrary conclusions were reached by Pim Cuijpers from the University of Amsterdam [27]. He accessed a database of 500 published randomized controlled trials of different psychotherapies for the treatment of depression in adults. The database was made up of trials of CBT, IPT, short-term psychodynamic psychotherapy, problem-solving therapy and other modalities.

Cuijpers concluded that psychotherapies are about equally as effective as medications and that combination treatments of psychotherapy with medications are more effective than either of these alone.

In comparing psychotherapy versus control groups, CBT had an effect size of 0.71. STPP effect size was 0.61. Both groups had significant heterogeneity.

The author concluded that overall the effect sizes from the different types of psychotherapy were not significantly different and that all of the therapies have comparable effects.

The conclusions of this vast study imply that common factors in psychotherapy are more important than specific factors. However the statistical power of the studies was too low to verify this. Large effect sizes were associated with the use of diagnostic criteria for depression, treatment manuals, therapist training and assessment of treatment integrity. Larger sample size, independent randomization, blind assessment of outcome and intention to treat analysis were also important factors [27].

4.6 Process Research

The aim of process research is to identify which treatment variables contribute to good outcomes. Patient characteristics determine 25–50% of the outcome variance. The therapeutic relationship accounts for 5–10% of the variance and therapist characteristics 8%. The specific method of psychotherapy used accounts for only 5–8% of the variance. These figures represent averages across a range of studies and methods. There is much room for improvement in treatment results. This will require answers to the question "which type of psychotherapy works best for which patients and with which problems?"

Process studies have identified the following key factors for effective therapeutic relationships: the working alliance, empathy, agreement on goals and collaboration.

Patient factors that influence therapy outcomes include functional impairment, patient expectations, attachment style and level of resistance.

These relationship factors cut across the different schools of psychotherapy. Process research supports transdiagnostic and trans-theoretical approaches to psychotherapy. However the evidence base is not as rigorous as that of randomized controlled trials focusing on specific disorders.

4.6.1 Common or Specific Factors: The Dodo Bird Effect

Based on current research findings, some authors have concluded that all forms of psychotherapy are about equally effective. This is known as the Dodo bird effect in reference to a character in Alice in Wonderland who stated that "everybody has won and all must have prizes" [28].

Jerome Frank in a widely acclaimed book identified common elements for all forms of psychotherapeutic methods [29]. He described six features that he felt were common to all psychotherapies:

- An intense, emotionally charged, confiding relationship with the helping person
- A rationale or myth which explains the cause of the patient's distress and a method for alleviating it
- The provision of new information concerning the patient's problems and possible alternative ways of dealing with them
- Strengthening the patient's expectations of help and the fostering of hope
- The provision of success experiences which increase the patient's hopes and enhance his sense of capability
- The facilitation of emotional arousal which is required for attitudinal and behavioural change

These six components have not lost their relevance during the intervening five decades since Frank described them. They are the focus of much current research.

Saul Rosenzweig may have been one of the first to bring attention to the importance of common factors in 1936 [30]. He ascertained that there are many implicit non-verbalized factors that lead to therapeutic change. He postulated that therapeutic results may be independent of specific theory as long as the theory is consistent. He recognized that different therapies may achieve change in different ways and different directions but could still lead to the required result because of the interrelationship of psychological variables. Theory and effectiveness do not have to be correlated.

Luborsky et al. found no difference in outcomes between different treatment models among 17 meta-analyses [31].

Messer and Wampold in a review of this controversy assert that common factors such as the therapeutic alliance and therapist characteristics account for most of the variance in treatment outcome equal to 5% to 7% of the variance [32].

4.7 Notable Studies of STPP

One of the most extensive and comprehensive meta-analyses of STPP was carried out by Abbass et al. in a Cochrane review. The authors undertook an extensive review of the literature, and based on selection criteria, 33 randomized controlled trials of short-term psychodynamic psychotherapy were selected for the meta-analysis [33]. Each study was rated on a range of criteria to estimate risk of bias at any stage in the trial process.

The trials were heterogeneous in nature and covered a range of diagnoses including depression, anxiety and a variety of somatic disorders. Overall results showed positive outcomes versus controls which included treatment as usual, waiting list controls or a comparator active treatment. The authors qualify their findings based on several methodological considerations. They concluded that short-term psychodynamic psychotherapy for 40 weeks or less may be effective for a range of common mental disorders with evidence of modest to large treatment effect sizes. The authors advised that the results should be interpreted with caution in view of the heterogeneity between studies and some loss of outcome significance at long-term follow-up.

Driessen, Abbass, Cuijpers and associates in 2015 updated a previous meta-analysis of short-term psychodynamic psychotherapy for depression carried out by this group completed in 2010.

This entailed 54 studies of which 33 were randomized controlled trials representing 3946 subjects [34].

No significant differences were found between individual STPP and other psychotherapies at post-treatment ($d = -0.14$) and follow-up ($d = -0.06$) in analyses that were adequately powered to detect a clinically relevant difference. STPP was significantly more efficacious than other psychotherapies on anxiety measures at both post-treatment ($d = 0.35$) and follow-up ($d = 0.76$).

In another study Driessen et al. undertook a randomized controlled trial of 341 adults meeting diagnostic criteria for major depression; they compared the efficacy of cognitive behavioral therapy (CBT) and psychodynamic therapy [35, 36].

Patients were randomized to 16 sessions of individual manualized CBT or short-term psychodynamic supportive psychotherapy. Severely depressed patients (HAM-D > 24) received additional antidepressant medication according to a protocol.

STPP was significantly more effective than control conditions at post-treatment on depression, general psychopathology and quality of life measures (d = 0.49–0.69). STPP pretreatment to post-treatment changes (d = 0.57–1.18) indicated significant improvements on all outcome measures, which either significantly improved further (d = 0.20–1.04) or were maintained from post-treatment to follow-up.

Steinert et al. performed a meta-analysis to test the equivalence of psychodynamic psychotherapy to other empirically supported treatments [37]. They selected 23 randomized controlled trials involving 2751 patients. They found that manual-guided psychodynamic therapy in adults was equivalent to other treatments with demonstrated efficacy.

In this study nonequivalence was statistically defined as the minimum difference that would be considered clinically significant between treatments. Twenty three randomized controlled trials published between 1983 and 2016 where included. Minimal sample size for each treatment was 20 in each group. The studies totalled 2751 patients. In most cases psychodynamic psychotherapy was compared with CBT. In two of the studies, the comparator was antidepressant medication. Studies varied in principal diagnosis. The authors concluded that psychodynamic therapy was as efficacious as other treatments including CBT.

Nevertheless the limitations of these and other meta-analysis have been pointed out.

The largest studies in Steinert's meta-analysis were those by Driessen et al. [35] and by Connolly Gibbons et al. [38].

Driessen's study compared 177 patients who received psychodynamic therapy with 164 patients who had CBT. Diagnosis was that of major depression with Hamilton Depression score greater than 14. Each group had 11 sessions. Outcomes were measured on the basis of symptoms.

Connolly Gibbons' trial compared 118 patients with psychodynamic therapy versus 119 patients with CBT each receiving 16 sessions of therapy for major depression. Outcomes included psychosocial functioning in addition to target symptoms. This study is notable for its relatively large sample size of 237 patients. Treatment was conducted at a single outpatient community mental health centre in Philadelphia, Pennsylvania.

The patients received 16 sessions of dynamic psychotherapy based on Luborsky's model. The Hamilton Depression rating scale was the primary outcome measure. Remission rates in both groups were only 22%.

The study found that dynamic therapy was not inferior to cognitive therapy in decreasing depressive symptoms. However it should be noted that there was no inactive control condition. The absence of a control group and the fact that 78% of participants did not respond to either treatment means improvement could be attributed to the passage of time.

4.8 The National Health Service

It is important also to consider the level of evidence required when discussing healthcare systems and funded services. The National Health Service in the United Kingdom has pioneered the provision of psychological services. Based on the National Institute for Healthcare Excellence (NICE) guidance, the NHS implemented a programme entitled "Improving Access to Psychological Therapies" (IAPT) in 2008.

Pybis et al. compared the outcomes of cognitive behavioural therapy and counselling in over 30,000 patients [39]. The principal outcome measures were the PHQ 9 and the

GAD 7. The authors undertook a multilevel analysis that considered number of sessions, baseline severity and the location at which the services were delivered.

The majority of patients suffered from depressive or anxiety disorders. "Reliable and clinically significant improvement" was defined as a reduction in PHQ 9 scores of 6 points or more. The mean number of sessions attended was 8.5 with a median of 7.

For CBT 46.6% of patients made reliable improvement. For those who had received generic counselling, 44.3% improved. There are no comparison data for other jurisdictions. These results appear to be good with the strong caveat that there was no randomization or blind ratings.

Even so 55% of patients did not improve leaving a need to identify more effective treatment approaches.

Therapy type was not a significant predictor of change. There was significant variability across treatment sites controlling for patient variables and number of sessions attended. It was not possible to measure therapist variables and to completely account for possible variations in case complexity.

4.9 Future Research

How can the quality of future of research be improved? Kocsis and colleagues have developed a 25-item questionnaire, the Randomized Controlled Trial of Psychotherapy Quality Rating Scale (RCT-PQRS) [40]. Items are rated on a 0 to 2 scale. The items rated include:

- Criteria for inclusion and exclusion.
- Diagnostic methods.
- Definition of the treatment used and how it is delivered. This requires review of transcripts or tapes, therapist training and experience and therapist supervision.
- Description of concurrent treatments.
- Use of validated outcome measures that are rated blindly.

- Assessment of post-termination long-term outcome following the end of the therapy.
- Use of the intent-to-treat method for data analysis.
- Adequate sample size.
- Comparison groups should be from the same population and studied within the same timeframe.

Using this rating scale, 94 randomized controlled trials of psychodynamic psychotherapy published between 1974 and 2010 were examined. Sixty-three of these studies were rated as having adequate quality. Thirty-nine studies included an active comparison treatment. A total sample size of at least 250 was estimated to yield enough power to detect differences between the experimental group and the active comparator. Smaller sample sizes are unable to detect the degree of difference sufficiently to establish a finding of "no difference". If the sample is large enough, then a finding of no difference between treatment methods indicates equal efficacy.

The same group of authors applied the same rating scale (RCT-PQRS) to assess the quality of randomized controlled trials of cognitive behavioural therapy for depression [41, 42].

One hundred and twenty randomized controlled trials of CBT were selected. It was possible to compare the quality rating score in 113 of these and 87 psychodynamic therapy studies. There was no significant difference in the psychodynamic and CBT quality scores. CBT trials had a mean quality rating of 25.5 with a standard deviation of 9.13. Psychodynamic trials had a mean quality rating of 25.1 and standard deviation of 9.04.

Studies rated with low quality were associated with an inflated outcome with larger effect sizes. Lower quality was also related to greater variability in outcomes. There is thus an inverse relationship between methodological quality and effect size. This may indicate that higher quality studies produce more valid results. It is important to note that the quality of the studies in both groups improved over time between 1975 and 2010.

The regular use of the RCT-PQRS could help to improve the quality of psychotherapy research in general and STPP research in particular. Optimal standards for psychodynamic research should include [41, 42]:

- Randomized controlled trials with adequate sample sizes.
- A manualized approach.
- Adequately trained therapists in the same method.
- Oversight to ensure fidelity to the method. The ideal would be video recordings of sessions.
- Valid outcome measures in all dimensions: symptomatic, functional, relational and subjective.
- Trials should include two control conditions: the first control condition, requires an active validated therapy in which the same standards are met (adequate sample size, adequate training of therapists, fidelity measures and adherence to a treatment manual). The second control condition would comprise of no active treatment such as weekly check-in meetings with a non-therapist or the completion of rating scales.

Key Points

- Randomized controlled trials and meta-analyses are considered the gold standards for conducting research on treatment outcome.
- Psychotherapy research involves particular difficulties in meeting all methodological requirements.
- Sample sizes, heterogeneity, fidelity to treatment models and therapist training are critical factors.
- Diagnostic homogeneity may be difficult to achieve.
- Biases include reporting bias, publication bias and allegiance bias.
- Much of the literature for all forms of psychotherapy do not meet adequate levels of quality.
- The best available evidence is that psychodynamic psychotherapy demonstrates positive outcomes in comparison to no treatment or treatment as usual. In head-to-head studies with active treatment, it may be equivalent.

- Larger randomized controlled trials using the same methods and populations are required and need to be replicated by different research groups to definitively demonstrate treatment effectiveness.
- STPP has demonstrated effectiveness in a range of psychiatric disorders including depression and anxiety in comparison to treatment as usual or inactive treatment.
- In comparison to proven active treatment such as cognitive behavioural therapy, the evidence points to equivalence, but this is a less robust finding at this point.
- The debate regarding the role of common and specific factors in the effectiveness of psychotherapy has not been resolved.
- Research should continue to identify better indications for specific therapy types.
- A distinction should be made between therapies that are primarily symptom orientated and those that are directed at changes in relational variables.

References

1. Haynes RB. Of studies, syntheses, synopses, summaries, and systems: the "5S" evolution of information services for evidence-based healthcare decisions. Evid Based Med. 2006;11(6):162–4.
2. Murad MH, Montori VM, Ioannidis JP, Jaeschke R, Devereaux PJ, Prasad K, Neumann I, Carrasco-Labra A, Agoritsas T, Hatala R, Meade MO, Wyer P, Cook DJ, Guyatt G. How to read a systematic review and meta-analysis and apply the results to patient care: users' guides to the medical literature. JAMA. 2014;312(2):171–9. https://doi.org/10.1001/jama.2014.5559.
3. Guyatt G. How to read a systematic review and meta-analysis and apply the results to patient care: users' guides to the medical literature. JAMA. 2014; 312(2):171–9. https://doi.org/10.1001/jama.2014.5559.

4. APA Presidential Task Force on Evidence-Based Practice. Evidence-based practice in psychology. Am Psychol. 2006;61(4):271–85.
5. Ioannidis JP. Why most published research findings are false. PLoS Med. 2005;2(8):0696–701.
6. Popper K. Conjectures and refutations: the growth of scientific knowledge. 5th ed. London: Routledge; 1989.
7. Lilienfeld SO. Introduction to special section on pseudoscience in psychiatry. Can J Psychiatr. 2015;60(12):531–3.
8. Meshikhes AN. Evidence-based surgery: the obstacles and solutions. Int J Surg. 2015;18:159–62.
9. Ulberg R, Ness E, Dahl HS, Høglend PA, Critchfield K, Blayvas P, Amlo S. Relational interventions in psychotherapy: development of a therapy process rating scale. BMC Psychiatry. 2016;16(1):310. https://doi.org/10.1186/s12888-016-1021-4.
10. Ulberg R, Amlo S, Høglend P. Manual for transference work scale: a micro-analytical tool for therapy process analyses. BMC Psychiatry. 2014;14:291. https://doi.org/10.1186/s12888-014-0291-y.
11. Høglend P. Exploration of the patient-therapist relationship in psychotherapy. Am J Psychiatry. 2014;171(10):1056–66. https://doi.org/10.1176/appi.ajp.2014.14010121.
12. Ulberg R, Amlo S, Critchfield KL, Marble A, Høglend P. Transference interventions and the process between therapist and patient. Psychotherapy (Chic). 2014;51(2):258–69. https://doi.org/10.1037/a0034708.
13. Hersoug AG, Høglend P, Gabbard GO, Lorentzen S. The combined predictive effect of patient characteristics and alliance on long-term dynamic and interpersonal functioning after dynamic psychotherapy. Clin Psychol Psychother. 2013;20(4):297–307. https://doi.org/10.1002/cpp.1770.
14. Høglend P, Hersoug AG, Bøgwald KP, Amlo S, Marble A, Sørbye Ø, Røssberg JI, Ulberg R, Gabbard GO, Crits-Christoph P. Effects of transference work in the context of therapeutic alliance and quality of object relations. J Consult Clin Psychol. 2011;79(5):697–706. https://doi.org/10.1037/a0024863.
15. Johansson P, Høglend P, Hersoug AG. Therapeutic alliance mediates the effect of patient expectancy in dynamic psychotherapy. Br J Clin Psychol. 2011;50(3):283–97. https://doi.org/10.1348/014466510X517406.
16. Høglend P, Dahl HS, Hersoug AG, Lorentzen S, Perry JC. Long-term effects of transference interpretation in dynamic psychother-

apy of personality disorders. Eur Psychiatry. 2011;26(7):419–24. https://doi.org/10.1016/j.eurpsy.2010.05.006.
17. Kallestad H, Valen J, McCullough L, Svartberg M, Høglend P, Stiles TC. The relationship between insight gained during therapy and long-term outcome in short-term dynamic psychotherapy and cognitive therapy for cluster C personality disorders. Psychother Res. 2010;20(5):526–34. https://doi.org/10.1080/10503307.2010.492807.
18. Hersoug AG, Høglend P Havik OE, Monsen JT. Development of working alliance over the course of psychotherapy. Psychol Psychother. 2010;83(Pt 2):145–59. https://doi.org/10.1348/147608309X471497.
19. Hersoug AG, Høglend P, Havik OE, von der Lippe A, Monsen JT. Pretreatment patient characteristics related to the level and development of working alliance in long-term psychotherapy. Psychother Res. 2009;19(2):172–80. https://doi.org/10.1080/10503300802657374.
20. Hersoug AG, Høglend P. Havik O, von der Lippe A, Monsen J. Therapist characteristics influencing the quality of alliance in long-term psychotherapy. Clin Psychol Psychother. 2009;16(2):100–10. https://doi.org/10.1002/cpp.605.
21. Høglend P, Bøgwald KP, Amlo S, Marble A, Ulberg R, Sjaastad MC, Sørbye O, Heyerdahl O, Johansson P. Transference interpretations in dynamic psychotherapy: do they really yield sustained effects? Am J Psychiatry. 2008;165(6):763–71. https://doi.org/10.1176/appi.ajp.2008.07061028.
22. McCullogh L, Kuhn N, Andrews, et al. Treating affect phobia a manual for short term dynamic psychotherapy. New York: Guilford press; 2003.
23. Gupta M. Is evidence-based psychiatry ethical? Oxford: Oxford University Press; 2014.
24. Cuthbert BN. Research domain criteria: toward future psychiatric nosologies. Dialogues Clin Neurosci. 2015;17(1):89–97.
25. Dragioti E, Karatnanos V, Gerdle B, Evangelou E. Does psychotherapy work? An umbrella review of meta-analyses of randomized controlled trials. Acta Psychiatr Scand. 2017;136:236–46.
26. Scott J. The science and practice of psychotherapy: the critical need for quality assurance and vigilance to monitor and the ratio of benefits to risks of therapies. Acta Psychiatr Scand. 2017;136:233–5.

27. Cuijpers P. Four decades of outcome research on psychotherapies for adult depression: an overview of a series of meta-analyses. Can Psychol/Psychologie Canadienne. 2017;58:7–19.
28. Carroll L. Alice's adventures in wonderland. London: Oxford University Press; 1971.
29. Frank JD, Frank J. Persuasion and healing: a comparative study of psychotherapy. 3rd ed. Baltimore: John Hopkins University Press; 1991.
30. Rosenzweig S. Some implicit common factors in diverse methods of psychotherapy. Am J Psychiatr. 1936;6:412–5.
31. Luborsky L, Rosenthal R, Diguer L, Andrusyna TP, Berman JS, Levitt JT, Seligman DA, Krause ED. The Dodo bird verdict is alive and well – mostly. Clin Psychol Sci Pract. 2002;9(1):2–12.
32. Messer SB, Wampold BE. Let's face facts: common factors are more potent than specific therapy ingredients. Clin Psychol Sci Pract. 2002;9(1):18–22.
33. Abbass AA, Kisely SR, Town JM, Leichsenring F, Driessen E, De Maat S, Gerber A, Dekker J, Rabung S, Rusalovska S, Crowe E. Short-term psychodynamic psychotherapies for common mental disorders. Cochrane Database of Systematic Reviews 2014, Issue 7. No.: CD004687. John Wiley & Sons. https://doi.org/10.1002/14651858.CD004687.pub4.
34. Driessen E, Hegelmaier LM, Abbass AA, Barber JP, Dekker JJ, Van HL, Jansma EP, Cuijpers P. The efficacy of short-term psychodynamic psychotherapy for depression: a meta-analysis update. Clin Psychol Rev. 2015;42:1–15. https://doi.org/10.1016/j.cpr.2015.07.004.
35. Driessen E, Van HL, Don FJ, et al. The efficacy of cognitive behavioral therapy and psychodynamic therapy in the outpatient treatment of major depression: a randomized clinical trial. Am J Psychiatr. 2013;170:1041–50.
36. Driessen E, Van HL, Peen J, Don FJ, Twisk JWR, Cuijpers P, Dekker JM. Cognitive-behavioral versus psychodynamic therapy for major depression: secondary outcomes of a randomized clinical trial. J Consult Clin Psychol. 2017;85:653–63. https://doi.org/10.1037/ccp0000207.
37. Steinert C, Munder T, Rabung S, Hoyer J, Leichsenring D. Psychodynamic therapy: as efficacious as other empirically supported treatments? A meta-analysis testing equivalence of outcomes. Am J Psychiatr Online. https://doi.org/10.1176/ajp.2017.17010057.

38. Connelly Gibbons MB, Gallup R, Thompson D, et al. Comparative effectiveness of cognitive therapy and dynamic psychotherapy for major depressive disorder in a community mental health setting: a randomized clinical noninferiority trial. JAMA Psychiatr. 2016;73:904–11.
39. Pybis J, Saxon D, Hill A, Barkham M. The comparative effectiveness and efficiency of cognitive behaviour therapy and generic counselling in the treatment of depression: evidence from the 2nd UK National Audit of psychological therapies. PMC Psychiatr. 2017;17:215.
40. Kocsis JH, Gerber AJ, Milrod B, Roose SP, Thase ME, Perkins P, Leon AC. A new scale for assessing the quality of randomized clinical trials of psychotherapy. Compr Psychiatry. 2010;51:319–24.
41. Thoma N, McKay D, Gerber A, Milrod B, Edwards A, Kocsis J. A quality- based review of randomized controlled trials of cognitive – behavioral therapy for depression: an assessment and meta-regression. Am J Psychiatr. 2012;169:22–30.
42. Gerber AJ, Kocsis JH, Milrod B, Roose SP, Barber J, Thase ME, Perkins P, Leon AC. A quality- based review of randomized controlled trials of psychodynamic psychotherapy. Am J Psychiatr. 2011;168(1):19–28.

Chapter 5
Updating the Language of Psychodynamic Psychotherapy

5.1 Background

The vocabulary of psychodynamic psychotherapy is rich and expressive. It originates from many different schools of psychodynamic theory each with its own spin on terminology: classical instinctual conflict theory of Freud; object relations theory of Melanie Klein, Donald Fairbairn, Michael Balint and Donald Winnicott; Kohut's self-psychology; and combinations of instinctual and object relations such as Edith Jacobson and Otto Kernberg. New terms have been added more contemporaneously from Bowlby's attachment theory, relational psychoanalysis and emotion-focused psychotherapies.

Yet there is a large lexicon of psychodynamic terminology that is shared across the various schools and systems. A shared conceptual repertoire may appear divided by terminological nuances. If psychodynamic psychotherapy continues to develop and be relevant, it must update its terminology to incorporate contemporary advances in affective and cognitive neurosciences. It must discard or modify terminology derived from theories that have been superseded by new models of psychological and interpersonal dynamics.

A. Eppel, *Short-Term Psychodynamic Psychotherapy*, https://doi.org/10.1007/978-3-319-74995-2_5

Very fundamentally we are still stuck with the mind-brain problem. Neurobiological research has been based on neurological lesion studies, animal studies and neuroimaging (Chap. 3). All of these lead to the conclusion that the experience of emotion, consciousness and human attachment, the very essence of the human experience, is derived from our neural circuits, neurons and synapses.

In this chapter some of the fundamental concepts and ideas that are generally utilized by experienced psychodynamic therapists are defined. Where the terminology is obscure or peculiar to a particular school of psychodynamic thought, a translation is proposed.

5.2 Definitions

5.2.1 Psychodynamics

This term conveys a sense of opposing forces. It is an active rather than static process. It implies interaction rather than disengagement. The word arises from Freud who used it to describe an interplay of forces in opposition to each other. To translate this into current paradigms, we might say that dynamics refers to cognitive and emotional processes that are constantly changing and reacting to internal and external stimuli. In particular, there is a dynamic interaction between the patient and the therapist.

5.2.2 Object Relations

The term object can lead to some confusion. Its use in psychodynamics comes from Freud and the German word "objekt". In psychodynamics it does not refer to "a thing" but to a person. The use of this word can only be understood by reference to Freudian instinct theory. For Freud instincts had "aims". The person towards whom the instinctual aim was directed or attracted to was termed "the object". For example, the sexual instinct may be directed towards a specific person who is described as "the object of the instinct" [1]. Similarly the target of a person's affection is termed a "love object". To avoid perplexity, it may be time to replace the word "object" with "other person".

Object relationship refers to an inner representation of interactions between two people: the self-representation and the object representation. An individual's ways of interacting with others depend on multiple differing internalized self-object interactions.

Donald Winnicott stressed that the formation of a sense of self depended on the interaction between the child and the environment. In this respect Winnicott is the forerunner of Bowlby's attachment theory. He theorised that the environment shapes the infant's development. The mother or mother substitute is the principal component of the environment in the early years of development. The term "good-enough mother" refers to the provision of sufficient caring, responsiveness and nurturance in order to ensure healthy development. This requires that the mother figure is responsive to differing needs that arise as the infant develops.

In the early stages of development, the infant is not aware of the boundary between himself and the external world. In Winnicott's terms, the infant has not yet differentiated the "me" from the "not me". In an adequately responsive environment, the infant develops a sense of himself. If the environment is not safe and the needs of the infant are not optimally met, this may lead to the development of "a false self". The false self masks the inner true self as a means of protection against a hostile or unloving environment. In adults a false self results in a lack of access to authentic inner emotions. The person is emotionally detached, "unreal" and unable to form meaningful relationships.

Transitional object is a term conceived by Winnicott to describe an area of experience between the inner mental world and the external world. This is an area where "me" and "not me" intersect. The words "transitional object" are universally recognized in describing a child's choice of a blanket or a soft toy from which he is inseparable. This object represents the mother or mother figure and stands in for her when she is not available to comfort the child. Transitional space includes those mental experiences that contain a mixture of inner reality and the external world. Aspects of play and culture represent transitional phenomena. For example, a painting contains representations of external reality but also contains aspects of the artist's own personality and inner reality.

One of the key functions of "good-enough mothering" is to convey to the infant that he is seen and recognized. This is a process of mirroring and responding. When this happens, when the infant is seen, his existence is confirmed.

"Holding environment" is the environment and atmosphere created by the mother that ensures the infants' safety and survival. It is characterised by predictability, acceptability and empathic responsiveness.

5.2.3 *Affect, Emotion and Feeling*

One of the thorniest problems in psychotherapeutics is to develop a consistent definition of the terms "affect", "emotion" and "feeling" (Chap. 3). Affect and emotion are often used interchangeably to describe biologically hardwired, genetically programmed processes that are experienced as visceral "in the gut". Wherever possible I have used the word emotion instead of affect in this book.

Emotions are made up of physiological, physical, psychological and hormonal patterns. They are intrinsically linked to preparatory physical states and actions. They arise from subcortical neurocircuits.

Feeling is often defined as the conscious experience of affect or emotion. Feelings arise from the cognitive perception and appraisal of emotions in areas of the neocortex.

Emotions can be classified into two main groups: adaptive and inhibitory. Adaptive emotions facilitate a healthy relationship with the external environment and consist of:

- Sadness/sorrow/grief
- Anger/irritation/rage/assertiveness/mastery
- Fear
- Happiness/joy/pride
- Attachment/love/compassion/care
- Sexual desire/lust

Inhibitory emotions tend to shut down adaptive behaviours leading to withdrawal and avoidance.

They include shame, humiliation and embarrassment which are activated in response to behaviour that is unacceptable to one's sense of self and society.

Guilt and self-blame are inhibitory and arise in response to behaviour that breaches social, family and cultural norms. Disgust and contempt inhibit attachment and closeness. Depression and mania are pathological emotional states which are qualitatively different from normal emotions.

5.3 Defences

A defence is psychological operation automatically and unconsciously deployed when an individual is facing a psychological threat. Defences protect the person by keeping certain thoughts and feelings out of awareness.

In Freudian conflict theory, the threat is from internal drives and impulses (aggressive, sexual) that threaten the ego resulting in anxiety. In object relations theory, the threat arises out of interactions with other people. Defences serve to keep the undesirable feelings related to a self or object representation out of awareness.

Interpersonal threats may threaten one's self-esteem or sense of identity. Threats may come from external events, dangers or losses. Threats may be to bodily integrity such as illness or injury. Defences are described as adaptive when they enhance functioning. Defences are maladaptive when they lead to impaired functioning, problems in relationships or symptoms.

Denial: sensory information regarding unpleasant external events is kept out of awareness.

Projection: inner feelings, impulses and thoughts are experienced as belonging to another person.

Projective identification: this consists of projection with the addition that the other person begins to behave and feel in accordance with what has been projected.

Splitting: self and other people are experienced as all good or all bad. This may shift back and forth.

Idealization: attributing to another person superior characteristics. Idealization provides the patient with a sense that they are going to be taken care of by an all-knowing and all-powerful attachment figure. Devaluation is the converse in which the person is experienced as disappointing, incompetent and of no value.

Somatization: the individual focuses on physical sensations to the exclusion of painful emotions.

Acting out: feelings are expressed through action rather than words.

Identification: unconsciously taking on characteristics, behaviours, attitudes and mannerisms of another person.

Displacement: the unconscious redirection of feelings associated with one person on to another.

Rationalization: providing logical explanations or excuses for unacceptable feelings, attitudes or behaviours.

Intellectualization: avoidance of feelings by focusing on logical and cognitive explanations.

Isolation of affect: separating thoughts from their associated emotions.

Reaction formation: the transformation of unacceptable feelings, wishes or impulses into their opposite.

Repression: the exclusion from awareness of feelings, thoughts or impulses arising internally.

Undoing: an attempt to neutralize unacceptable aggressive, sexual or shameful feelings by elaborating contradictory behaviours or thoughts.

Controlling: distraction from feelings by means of control, organization and regimentation of tasks and other people.

Sexualisation: focuses on sexual aspects of another person defending against the experience of painful emotions.

Dissociation: alteration in the awareness of current events, surroundings and time in the presence of full consciousness.

Humour: the automatic unconscious use of humour to divert focus from unpleasant feelings.

Humour may represent the disguised expression of feelings without personal discomfort and may conceal feelings or behaviours that are unacceptable to others.

Sarcasm: the expression of anger disguised as humour.

Passive aggression: the indirect expression of aggression through deniable behaviours such as lateness, procrastination, forgetting to do things and inconveniencing others.

Externalization: the attribution of the responsibility for one's feelings or behaviours to external factors or people.

Altruism: behaviour is directed towards the needs of others rather than to one's own needs and desires.

Sublimation: the unconscious diversion of emotions, desires and behaviours into socially productive activities.

Masochism: self-sacrifice of one's own needs, wishes and gratifications as a defence against feelings of guilt, shame or anger.

It should be emphasised that defences are not the same as "coping mechanisms". Coping mechanisms are consciously deployed to reduce distressing emotions and thoughts.

Coping mechanisms include conscious suppression of thoughts, feelings and behaviours. The coping strategy of anticipation entails postponing immediate gratification of feelings and wishes in the expectation of future benefits. The conscious as opposed to unconscious use of humour is also a coping mechanism.

5.3.1 Neuroscientific Reformulation of Concept of Defence

Defence mechanisms can be understood in terms of the Dual Processing model of emotion (Chap 3).

External physical threats trigger an appraisal by the organism and a fight or flight response. This involves the activation of various control centres including the autonomic nervous system, the attentional and motor systems.

Psychological threats are triggered by internal or external stimuli that undergo fast or slow appraisal by means of either the subcortical low road or the cognitive high road. Strategies employed at the cognitive level are more correctly called coping strategies that are made on a conscious basis.

Defence mechanisms operate on the low road and occur automatically leading to activation of different behavioural and emotional responses; certain outputs are activated while others are inhibited. This must be mediated through a control centre that computes the values of the alternative responses. If safety is restored, the computation changes in value and may allow the individual to risk vulnerability and disclose feelings. Therapeutic interventions are designed to enhance safety and reduce defences thereby permitting emotional expression.

Transference is the re-experiencing of feelings towards another person based on internal working models. This leads to expectations and attributions which may not be accurate to the current interaction.

Countertransference comprises the transference feelings that the therapist has towards the patient which are determined by his or her own internal working models.

5.4 Attachment Theory, Object Relations and Interpersonal Terms

Internal working models develop in the early years of childhood based on attachment experiences. Internal working models are made up of multiple experiences of self in relation to others (Table 5.1). Self-representations consist of emotional, cognitive and physical attributes and are linked to representations of others. These self-other templates are linked by emotion, bodily feelings, cognitions and memories.

Table 5.1 Definition of attachment theory concepts

Proximity seeking	The genetic programme that causes infants to seek proximity to its mother
Separation anxiety	The distress experienced by an infant when separated from the primary attachment figure. Indicated by fear, crying and agitation
Secure base	The feeling of safety and security provided by the primary attachment figure that allows the infant to begin to separate and explore the world
Safe haven	The function provided by the secure base when the infant is in distress and seeks proximity to the attachment figure. Activation of this is brought about by separation, strangeness, pain, hunger, fatigue
Principal or Primary attachment figure (PAF)	This is the person who has the most day-to-day interaction with the infant. It may be a parent, grandparent, sibling or other caregiver
Internal working models	These are emotional and cognitive representations of the external world. They consist of representations of the self and representations of others. The early attachment relationships form the foundations for emotionally based representations of relationships with others

5.4.1 Translating Dynamic Terms into Attachment Language

It is possible to redefine psychodynamic terminology using attachment theory concepts (Table 5.2). I often use the analogy of Pythagoras' theorem which states that "in a right-angled triangle, the square of the hypotenuse is equal to the sum of the squares of the other two sides". This is rather cumbersome and archaic language. The same concept can be much more concisely and clearly expressed using the language of algebra (Fig. 5.1):

TABLE 5.2 Comparison of attachment and object relations concepts

Attachment theory	**Object relations**
Secure base	Therapeutic alliance
Exploration	Capacity to be alone
Internal working models	Self- and object representations
Attunement	Holding environment
Attachment style	Defences
Mentalization- existing in the heart and mind of the other	Reflective functioning
Implicit memory	Unconscious
Attachment relationships	Self and objects

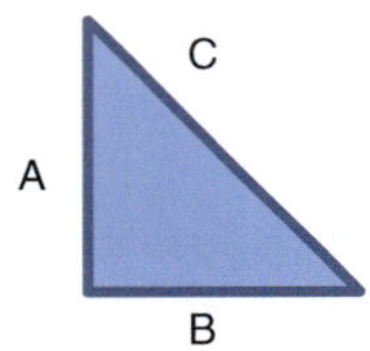

FIGURE 5.1 A Right-angle triangle

$A^2 + B^2 = C^2$ where C is the longest side of the triangle and A and B are the other two sides.

I compare the language of Euclidean geometry to that of many psychodynamic terms: very rich, descriptive, at times poetic and beautifully structured. However attachment theory, like algebra, is more consistent with contemporary science and for students easier to grasp.

5.5 Memory

There are two main categories of memory: explicit memory and implicit memory.

Explicit memory is also known as declarative memory and refers to memories that are conscious and available for recall.

Declarative memory stores specific facts, events, people's names, places and information.

There are two subcategories for explicit memory:

Autobiographical (episodic) and semantic memory.

Autobiographical memory consists of events connected to a specific time and place. It includes memories of oneself as a participant in the event. Autobiographical memories provide a sense of continuity and hence identity. Autobiographical memory includes the memory of associated feelings.

Semantic memory consists of general knowledge, facts and meanings of words and data that are not attached to specific times or places.

Implicit memory operates outside of awareness and encompasses procedural memory. Procedural memory is also known as non-declarative memory.

Procedural memory refers to actions that are carried out automatically. They do not involve consciousness. An example of this is riding a bicycle, the memories of which are stored in the basal ganglia and cerebellum. Relationship patterns depend on implicit relational knowledge and generally unfold automatically.

5.6 Empathy

Empathy has also been described as biographical, semantic and procedural [2].

Procedural empathy is synonymous with emotional contagion and refers to the automatic synchronization of facial emotions between two people. This form of empathy is unconscious and appears to be inborn. An example of this is yawning. This appears to be dependent on visual and motor neural circuits (Fig. 5.2).

Semantic empathy is expressed verbally. It is the ability to consciously identify, recognize and name facial emotions (top-down).

Figure 5.2 Empathy

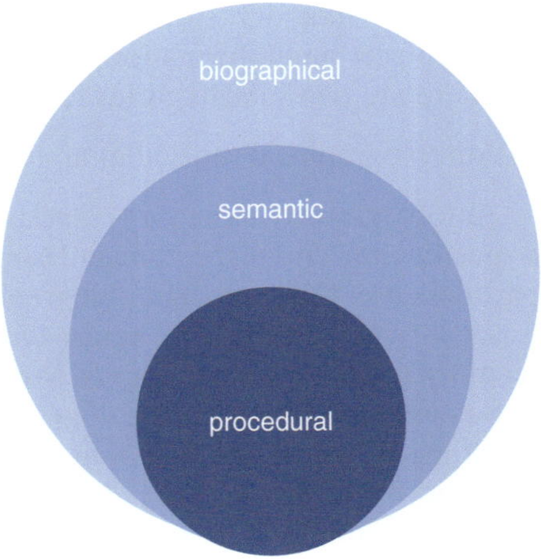

Biographical empathy draws on personal life experience and has emotional and verbal components.

Projective identification may in fact represent procedural empathy.

Empathy involves both sharing of emotions and being able to understand the other person's point of view. The latter requires the activation of the therapist's own mental representations and memories.

Empathy can thus be viewed as the activation of the therapist's own personal neural circuits and mental representations of the state that is being observed. This can be referred to as emotional empathy as opposed to cognitive empathy which is a deliberative top-down activation. Cognitive empathy entails consciously "stepping into the other's shoes". It is a process of imagination and deliberate recall of associated memories.

5.7 Therapeutic Change Processes

This refers to the processes that bring about changes in symptoms, self-other representations/ internal working models and relationship patterns.

Lane et al. propose that therapeutic change results from a three-step process [3].

- Reactivating old memories
- Engaging in new emotional experiences that are then incorporated into the reactivated memories by reconsolidation
- Reinforcing the changed memory structure by practising new ways of behaving in multiple contexts [3]

This requires optimal arousal of emotion in therapy sessions in accordance with the Goldilocks rule (Chap. 6).

5.8 Statistical Language

5.8.1 Meta-analysis

Meta-analysis is a statistical procedure that is used when individual randomized control trials are not large enough to make valid conclusions. The process of meta-analysis is a mathematical procedure that combines the results of multiple individual studies [4, 5].

The detailed procedures of carrying out a meta-analysis are beyond the scope of this book. The calculations can be done by specific software programmes.

The results of a meta-analysis are displayed in a "forest plot". This is a graphical display in which all of the individual trials are listed on the left-hand side.

Results are displayed in horizontal lines that contain point estimates and a 95% confidence interval. The confidence interval is an estimate of the range in which the true effect size lies in the population of interest.

5.8.2 Effect Size

Effect size is a standardized measure that allows comparison of results from different studies. Effect sizes are the most important outcome measures in psychotherapy research studies.

Cohen's d is a commonly used effect size in psychotherapy research. Cohen's d is calculated from the mean differences of an effect. An effect size is considered small if $d = 0.2$, medium if $d = 0.5$ and large if $d = 0.8$. However these values are arbitrary and should be related to the clinical impact of the findings.

An alternative measure is Hedge's g. Population effect sizes are estimated on the basis of the study samples and may overestimate the true population effect. The calculation of Hedges g is used to correct for this bias particularly when sample sizes are small.

Another group of effect sizes is based on correlation and indicated by the letter r.

5.8.3 Heterogeneity

Heterogeneity refers to the level of differences between studies included in the meta-analysis. There may be differences in inclusion criteria for patients in the study. There may be differences in measures of outcome and other methodological differences. This is the proverbial problem of comparing apples and oranges! Measures must be employed to determine if the level of heterogeneity is too high which would indicate that the results of the meta-analysis are not valid. It is important to check for measures of heterogeneity when appraising the results of a meta-analysis.

Key Points

- The language of psychodynamics is based on multiple theories and schools of thought.
- Concepts need to be redefined to take into account advances in affective and cognitive neurosciences.
- Defences can be conceptualized as implicit emotion regulation systems.

- Effect size is a standardized measure that allows comparison of results from different studies.
- Effect sizes are the most important outcome measures in psychotherapy research studies.

References

1. Laplanche J, Pontalis J-B. The language of psychoanalysis. London: Karnac; 2006.
2. Guilé JM. Disentangling cognitive processes from neural activation and psychic mechanisms: the example of empathy. J Physiol. 2010;104:337–41.
3. Lane RD, Ryan L, Nadel L, Greenberg L. Memory reconsolidation, emotional arousal, and the process of change in psychotherapy: new insights from brain science. Behav Brain Sci. 2015;38:e1. https://doi.org/10.1017/S0140525X14000041.
4. Hak T, Van Rhee HJ, Suurmond R. How to interpret results of meta-analysis. (Version 1.0). Rotterdam: Erasmus Rotterdam Institute of Management; 2016. www.erim.eur.nl/research-support/meta-essentials/downloads.
5. Greenhalgh T. How to read a paper: the basics of evidence-based medicine. 5th ed. Chichester: Wiley; 2014.

Chapter 6
Choice Point Analysis and Action Alternatives

6.1 Background

The fundamental process in psychodynamic therapy consists of a back and forth interactive dialogue between the therapist and the patient: the patient speaks; the therapist listens; the therapist speaks; the patient responds. What the therapist says is an "intervention".

At any instant during a therapy session, the therapist has to choose from multiple possible interventions.

These are "choice points" and "action alternatives". Lewis Tauber describes a choice point as "a critical point requiring action on the part of the therapist" [1]. Tauber called his system "choice point analysis". The options or choices which are available to the therapist are referred to by Tauber as "action alternatives".

This model involves the therapist considering what would be the most effective intervention at any moment in the therapeutic process. The therapist must consider which of the options will best facilitate the flow of therapy at each point.

A choice point occurs when there is a need for the therapist to make an intervention.

Examples where this need may be identified:

- The session is "not going anywhere".
- The content of the session is superficial and insignificant.
- The patient appears angry or withholding.

A. Eppel, *Short-Term Psychodynamic Psychotherapy*, https://doi.org/10.1007/978-3-319-74995-2_6

- The patient confronts the therapist.
- The patient is disengaged.
- The patient displays an emotional shift.
- The therapist experiences an emotional shift.
- Silence.
- There is an intensification of anxiety in patient or therapist.

In order for the therapist to identify choice points and action alternatives, he must constantly track what the patient is saying, nonverbal cues, signs of emotion and his own responses to the patient. The therapist listens attentively and needs to pay attention to facial expressions, gesture, posture and tone of voice.

At a choice point, the therapist must opt to make an intervention. He has to decide to speak.

What should he say? Which interventions should the therapist make? Which interventions when applied over the course of treatment result in better outcomes?

How does the beginning therapist learn what to say and when to say it? To answer this question, I first review key ideas on clinical decision theory and then describe the method developed by Dr. Lewis Tauber when supervising trainee psychotherapists [1].

6.2 How Do We Make Decisions?

There is an extensive literature on decision-making processes. This has major relevance in many disciplines. The issue for the therapists and for teachers is whether clinical decisions can be based on rational choices as opposed to intuition. Psychologist Daniel Kahneman studied the decision-making process in Economics and found that this is not an exclusively cognitive procedure [2, 3]. He subsequently won the Nobel Prize in Economics for the development of his dual processing view of decision-making which entails two systems which he termed "System 1" and "System 2".

System 1 operates automatically and is the faster of the two systems, with "little or no awareness of effort and no sense of voluntary control" [3]. This is "intuitive" and non-analytic.

System 2 refers to a conscious reasoning process that makes choices and is associated with the "subjective experience of agency, choice and concentration". This appears to be similar to the ideas of conscious and unconscious, explicit or implicit thought processes in psychodynamics and psychology.

System 1 and System 2 are continuously active. System 1 constantly generates impressions, intuitions, tensions and feelings. System 2 may appraise these inputs and convert to voluntary behaviour. Similar concepts were elaborated by Metcalfe and Mischel which they described as "hot" and "cool" thinking [4].

Kahneman's theories have been applied to clinical decision-making in order to reduce error, to eliminate cognitive biases and to make diagnoses more accurate. The current consensus is that clinical reasoning and decision-making involve continuous interaction of both System 1 and System 2. Intuitive and deliberative processes work simultaneously.

System 1 processes are based on pattern recognition. This in turn depends on memories and prior experience. The expert is responding to a cue that triggers access to information stored in memory [3].

Studies by Geoff Norman and Jonathan Sherbino and others at McMaster University [5] have shown that experienced clinicians often rely more on System 1 processes then on analytical reasoning.

The results of their research have demonstrated that "gut feeling" plays an important role in clinical decision-making. This finding is surprising as it has long been thought that expert clinicians make decisions based on greater knowledge, the ability to utilize deductive reasoning and the application of rational diagnostic and treatment algorithms. Because of the role of System 1 in clinical work, the novice is often puzzled by a supervisor's ability to make more rapid decisions about diagnosis or treatment. Yet when novices rely on "gut feeling", it is more likely to lead to error [5].

The answer to this paradox is that gut feelings of the novice and gut feelings of the expert are very different. System 1 operates rapidly based on unconscious pattern recognition arising from experiential implicit memories acquired over many years. The student does not have this memory "bank" from which valid predictions are generated.

Kahneman [3] distinguishes true expert judgement from false confidence which produces an illusion of validity. The conditions for expert intuition require a body of knowledge that contains regular components that are predictable. It must be possible to acquire this knowledge through prolonged practice. Kahneman describes the game of chess as an example of a body knowledge that leads to regular and predictable results. The chessmaster relies on System 1 intuition when moving his chess pieces. Experts like chessmasters and seasoned physicians are able to respond to specific cues that trigger stored experiences and memories. This is in contrast to trying to predict the stock market in which the process lacks sufficient regularity! Intuition cannot be correct in an unpredictable environment. The environment must contain some stable regularities that can be learned [3].

With regard to psychotherapy, Kahneman notes that psychotherapists can develop expertise about the effect of in-session interventions. A psychotherapist is able to observe the immediate response of the patient, and this feedback results in learning and storage of memories. However psychotherapists are unable to make good predictions about long-term outcome because they receive insufficient feedback about this to influence their modes of practice. Short-term and long-term predictions depend on the environment and context. For example, physicians working in specialties in which they only see patients on one occasion will not be in a position to make longer-term predictions about new patients because they receive no long-term feedback about the outcomes of their treatment.

Without feedback longer-term predictions are based on lack of stored data and more prone to cognitive biases such as overgeneralisation.

Although Norman and Sherbino's studies [5] concern the diagnostic process, it is reasonable to extrapolate that System 1 and System 2 processes are at work when deciding to make a therapeutic intervention in psychotherapy. The therapist also has to make an appraisal ("diagnosis") and match this to the intervention that is most likely to be useful.

At this point we do not have extensive empirical evidence as to which intervention is the best at any one moment in time. There is substantial process research to guide us, but there is a need for future research and refinement. This in turn will help to answer what are the main research questions of psychotherapy: which intervention for which patients for which disorders? Unfortunately the answers to these questions are not readily available. Research is difficult. There is a need for large sample sizes, for therapists to have standardized training and manualized methods.

6.3 Lewis Tauber: Choice Points and Action Alternatives

Lewis Tauber developed a system for use in supervising trainee therapists which he called "choice point analysis" [1]. Tauber's concept of choice points distils the essence of the therapist's task. At any one moment during therapy, the therapist must consider more than a dozen or so possible interventions. The therapist must choose the most effective intervention in the therapy session to advance the goals of treatment. Tauber describes seven groups of "action alternatives". The following are ones that have relevance to individual psychotherapy:

I. Action alternatives

(i) Silence.
(ii) Pursue affect. This can be intensifying affect or down regulating affect.
(iii) Pursue content.

II. Direction alternatives

The therapist can direct his intervention towards the patient or towards himself.

III. Time alternatives

The therapist can choose the here and now, the past or the future to frame his intervention.

IV. Precision alternatives

The intervention may be general or specific. If general the intervention may refer to a group of people rather than specifically to the patient. The phrasing can be narrowed to achieve "surgical" precision.

V. Stance alternatives

The therapist's stance can be neutral, supportive and empathic, confrontational or directive.

VI. Focus alternatives

These refer to the therapist's objectives at a particular point. This includes collecting information, reflecting reality, producing insight or producing emotional release.

Tauber's aim was to teach the student to reflect on intervention alternatives and select the one that would promote the attainment of therapy goals. We can conceptualize this now as making *implicit* System 1-based decisions *explicit* and subject to System 2 decision-making.

Tauber supervised students in small groups. He felt one supervisor and three supervisees were optimal. He used videotaped recordings of the students' sessions. During the supervision, the recording is stopped at various points, and alternative actions are discussed. The use of alternative interventions could be demonstrated with role-playing. This assists the supervisees to determine which is the preferred intervention.

Since the time of Tauber's work, there has been an evolution of interventions in the field of psychodynamic psychotherapy (Chap. 1). Theories and techniques have been developed in the works of Gabbard [6, 7], Malan [8–10], Davanloo [11], Luborsky [12], Fosha [13], McCullogh [14], Abbass [15] and others.

The psychotherapy process literature identifies several interventions that correlate with positive outcome. Across all therapies the therapeutic alliance predicts a significant amount of the variance in treatment outcome. Other critical areas include interpretation of the transference, processing of affect, focusing on the relationship between the patient and the therapist, identifying ruptures in the relationship and undertaking repair.

6.3.1 AEDP and Fosha's Emphasis on the Dyad

Diana Fosha has evolved a vigorous but highly empathic emotional focus in accelerated experiential dynamic psychotherapy [13]. Fosha states that the unit of intervention is not the therapist's comment but the therapist's comment and the patient's response. It is the patient's experience of the intervention that determines its therapeutic impact. The therapist can make an empathic intervention, but it is necessary to explore whether or not the patient experiences it as empathic.

Fosha identifies three main groups of intervention [13]:

- Relational strategies which include the therapist's expression of support, affirmation and empathy. Relational interventions help get past defences. These interventions indicate collaboration such as "I am here to help","You are not alone" and "We are in this together. Fosha emphasizes the use of the word "we" to foster the attachment relationship and the shared nature of the therapeutic journey. Relational strategies include acknowledging and repair of ruptures, self-disclosure and acknowledgement of therapist errors.

  Fosha has highlighted the relational process of "metaprocessing". Metaprocessing is one of AEDP's most powerful contributions to the practice of STPP [13]. The dual processing model of emotion (Chap. 2) provides a neuroscientific rationale for effect this intervention has for therapeutic change. Metaprocessing involves reflecting on the experience of experiencing. It is the cognitive awareness of the "feeling" of emotions that have their origins in subcortical processes.

- By experiencing and processing core emotions in the therapy session, negative valences attached to specific memories can be altered. The memories are then reconsolidated without the negative emotional "tags".
- Restructuring strategies: identifying, labelling and clarification of defences. Pointing out the maladaptive aspects of defences and reinforcing alternatives.
- Experiential-affective strategies. These include helping the patient to become aware of deep emotions. It involves tolerating the experience of emotions in the present moment and staying with the emotion long enough to process it. Incidentally this strategy is consistent with McCullogh's view that exposure to emotion is a major therapy change factor [14].

The experience of emotion can be enhanced by amplifying techniques. These include focusing on the bodily experience of emotion and the use of portrayals: imagined interactions.

6.4 STPP Interventions

Moving beyond Tauber, we need to determine which interventions are utilized in short-term psychodynamic psychotherapy and which ones are associated with successful outcomes. Leichsenring and colleagues [16] have identified prototypical interventions the psychotherapy process Q-set. The PQS is a 100-item questionnaire used to rate an ideal therapy session. Experts in supportive-expressive psychotherapy, a form of STPP based on Luborsky's method, rated audiotapes and videotapes of sessions to determine and rank order the items that were most and least characteristic of supportive-expressive psychotherapy.

This study found that the following interventions were typical of therapists engaged in supportive-expressive therapy and psychoanalysis. Examples include:

- Identifying a recurrent theme
- Nonjudgemental acceptance and empathy
- Noting mood and feelings including those unacceptable to the patient [16]

The following interventions were among those used in supportive-expressive therapy but not by the psychoanalytic therapists [16]:

- Asking for information
- Discussing current life situation
- Addressing termination
- Discussing patient's interpersonal relationships
- Adopting a supportive stance
- Discussing patient's goals
- Explaining the rationale for the therapeutic approach
- Encouraging the patient's independence of action or opinion
- Addressing a specific focus
- Encouraging the patient to try new ways of behaving with others

This list of prototypical interventions provides a unique way to compare different forms of psychotherapies. This can more systematically identify overlapping techniques. The items detailed in the lists of interventions can be considered "action alternatives".

6.5 Evidence for Interventions and Treatment Outcomes

In order to select the priority choice points, it is necessary to examine which interventions are correlated with good treatment outcomes.

The research literature identifies a number of interventions that correlate with positive outcome.

Across all therapies, the therapeutic alliance accounts for a significant portion of the variance in treatment outcome. Therefore interventions promoting a good alliance should rate high on our list of choice points. Other critical areas include interpretation of the transference, processing of affect, focusing on the relationship between the patient and the therapist, identifying ruptures in the relationship and undertaking repair.

6.5.1 Promoting the Therapeutic Alliance

Horvath et al. reviewed over 200 studies involving 14,000 patients on the relationship between alliance and the outcomes of individual psychotherapy [17].

The overall effect size of 0.275 was statistically significant. Even though this only accounted for a small proportion of the total variance in treatment outcome, it is one of the strongest predictors of treatment success [17]. The therapeutic alliance in individual psychotherapy accounts for approximately 7.5% of the variance in treatment outcomes.

The development of a "good-enough" alliance early in therapy is vital for therapy success.

The therapeutic alliance can also be conceptualized in attachment terms. Bowlby (Chap. 2) postulated that the therapist provides "a secure base" for the patient. In early childhood development, the infant is able to explore its environment only after it has established a secure attachment and internalized a sense of a secure base.

Short-term dynamic psychotherapies including experiential dynamic therapy emphasize explicit therapeutic interventions to establish and deepen the therapeutic alliance.

Diana Fosha's relational interventions are very effective in establishing a secure attachment between patient and therapist [13]. The patient and the therapist's own attachment status will affect the development of the therapeutic alliance.

6.5.2 Emotion Focus

Exploring emotion is another prototypical item in STPP. It requires the therapist to help the patient to identify and express feelings that may have been avoided or which may be unconscious.

Diener [18] undertook a meta-analysis of 10 studies comprising of 150 subjects examining the relationship between outcome and the adoption of an affective focus. The authors found that this was positively associated with improvements in treatment. The overall effect size of $r = 0.30$ represents a medium effect size.

Ablon et al. [19] studied 17 patients with panic disorder treated by 7 psychodynamically orientated therapists at the Massachusetts General Hospital Psychiatry outpatient department. They used the psychotherapy process Q-set to rate audiotapes. These process measures were then correlated with outcome.

Interventions focusing on feelings had the highest association with positive outcome.

The item "Therapist emphasizes patient's feelings to deepen them" had a robust effect size of 0.70. The effect size for the item "Therapist draws attention to feelings patient regards as unacceptable' was 0.43. Interestingly the use of humour yielded a 0.52 effect size.

However it may not be possible to consider process measures as independent of each other. In a study of 101 patients attending a university outpatient clinic, Fisher [20] examined the interplay between emotional experience, therapeutic alliance and patient functioning. They found that a strong alliance and the experience of deep emotions act synergistically to improve the patients' functioning and wellbeing. McCarthy's paper [21] adds a further dimension of complexity to the story.

In a study of 33 patients randomized to treatment with psychodynamic psychotherapy for patients with major depressive disorder versus pharmacotherapy and placebo, McCarthy and co authors found that process variables had a curvilinear relationship to outcome. Too many or too few psychodynamic and process-experiential interventions were less effective than intermediate levels. They referred to this as the "Goldilocks effect".

6.5.3 Transference and Relationship

Identifying and working with the transference has been regarded as a sine qua non in all forms of psychodynamic psychotherapy. The concept of transference and countertransference is viewed as one of Freud's most important contributions to the field of psychoanalysis and psychotherapy. David Malan with colleagues at the Tavistock Clinic in London was among the first to systematically examine the impact of transference interpretations on treatment outcome [8–10]. In a series of studies, Malan found that the frequency of transference interpretations when linked to experiences with parents or siblings was associated with better treatment outcome.

Habib Davanloo [11] placed working with intense transference feelings at the heart of his method.

Marziali replicated Malan's findings on the outcome link to the frequency with which the therapist referred to emotions in the transference [22]. These interpretations connected the transference with similar emotions experienced towards parents and other important figures. Marziali used audiotapes of sessions from 25 patients unlike Malan who had used written transcripts.

The subsequent literature has demonstrated that the association between a focus on transference and outcome is not a straightforward linear relationship. In a series of in-depth studies carried out as part of the First Experimental Study of Transference (FEST) at the University of Oslo, Høglend and colleagues found that the impact of a transference interpretation is dependent on a number of other variables: the therapeutic alliance, the patient's quality of object relations, the number of transference interpretations per session and the timing [23, 24]. There was an interaction effect: the alliance had a significantly different impact on effects of transference interpretation, depending on the quality of object relations. The impact of transference interpretation on psychodynamic functioning was more positive within the context of a weak therapeutic alliance for patients with a low quality of object relations. For patients with more mature object relations and high alliance, the authors observed a negative effect of transference work. These findings run completely counter to the conventional view.

6.5.4 Rupture and Repair in the Relationship

Safran et al. found that a key to therapeutic change is negotiation of ruptures in the alliance [25,26]. Metacommunication, talking about what is being enacted in the therapeutic relationship, is critical. The focus is on "the here and now" rather than "the developmental origins of what is being enacted in the therapeutic relationship".

Safran identified two main types of rupture: withdrawal ruptures and confrontation ruptures. The therapist must have the skills to be able to identify that there has been a rupture. Then the patient's feelings need to explored and worked through.

Ruptures may be signalled by postural changes such as gaze aversion or crossing of the arms. Other indications include silence, interrupting, demanding, a sarcastic or mocking tone. Other more obvious signs include criticisms of the therapist's personality or competence.

Clara Hill also stresses the centrality of processing the therapeutic relationship [27]. Hill uses the term "relationship" to include the real relationship, the therapeutic alliance, transference and countertransference.

Processing involves working in the here and now, inquiring about reactions to the therapist, drawing parallels with other relationships, processing ruptures or boundary crossings and disclosing feelings of closeness to or lack of closeness from others. "Metacommunication" refers to this communication about the relationship and includes addressing feelings about each other.

Diana Fosha's method of accelerated experiential dynamic psychotherapy (AEDP) described above is consistent with the approaches taken by Hill and Safran. The use of self-disclosure about the patient's impact, acknowledging errors, repairing therapeutic ruptures and metaprocessing are all critical to the AEDP approach.

6.5.5 The Relational Focus

The central theme or relational focus is essential for guiding the therapy process. It provides coherence to interpretive interventions and is the fulcrum around which the patient becomes aware of his or her interpersonal patterns and the impact this has on relationships and emotions. The focus makes sense out of what is at first an amorphous mass of information that the patient brings to the therapeutic encounter. The use of a focus extracts key dynamic elements that reflect the patient's internal working models.

Working with the relational theme and the experience of a corrective emotional experience results in a change in the internal working models. STPP can be regarded as using the therapeutic relationship to remodel the attachment-based internal working models (Chap. 2).

Joyce and Piper [28] in a study of 60 cases using a manualized form of brief psychodynamic therapy found that interventions related to the focus had positive effects on therapy outcome. In the same study, however, they noted that a high frequency of transference interpretations had a negative impact for patients rated high on a scale of quality of object relations. This seems to imply that interventions relating to a focus are beneficial but that the use of transference interventions that are based on the focus can have an opposing affect.

Much of the work establishing the importance of a focus was done by Luborsky's group [29]. To be successful, the core focus should be linked to the patient's identified problems and goals.

I attempt to present a provisional focus within the first three to four sessions and give it in written form to the patient. The patient and the therapist should collaborate on the development of the relational focus based on the history of past and current relationship patterns and feelings about oneself. Over the course of therapy, the focus can be refined based on new emerging themes, memories and clarifications (Chap. 7).

The focus helps provide a frame of reference for the conduct of therapy and gives unity and coherence to a large amount of clinical information.

As with all of these choice points, it is artificial to separate process components without acknowledging that all of these interact with each other and that outcomes are not a linear or arithmetic combination of the required elements.

The psychotherapy process is not a closed system and involves multiply interactive and transactional variables.

6.5.6 *Humour*

Therapist variables have a significant impact on the course of therapy and its outcome. This includes the therapist's own personality characteristics and attachment style.

There is variation among therapist's ability to use humour. The impact of the use of humour on outcomes is infrequently studied. Nevertheless on the face of it, humour may contribute to a positive therapeutic alliance.

Some authors have pointed out that humour can potentially be harmful in psychotherapy [30]. There is a significant risk that the patient may feel that he is being laughed at, that he is being belittled or that his concerns are being trivialized or mocked. The therapist must be aware of how the humorous remark or joke will be received. This depends on the therapist having a good sense of the quality of the therapeutic alliance and the patient's vulnerability to feeling shamed.

Humour can be used judiciously if it is compatible with the therapist's own personality and with the patient's capacity to receive it. Valentine and Gabbard believe that the use of humour in therapy can be taught [31]. It may be helpful to make students aware of the risks, appropriateness and the limitations of humour in therapy.

There is some evidence that humour has a beneficial effect. Richman described situations where he felt that humour in therapy was helpful to patients with depression and suicidal thoughts. He felt that humour is life-affirming, reduces stress and promotes symptom relief and social cohesion [32].

There is interesting evidence from the advertising world that humour can have powerful implicit effects [33]. Humour in advertising appears to counteract negative associations to product brands.

In this study among university students in Nijmegen, Netherlands, these authors showed that humour prevented the development of negative brand associations. The effect of humour was more powerful than that of positive or neutral stimuli.

If we extrapolate these findings to psychotherapy, it may be hypothesized that humour can alter the negative valence associated with emotionally charged memories.

Humour can be used to challenge defences, to challenge the absurdity of patient's self-blame or feelings of guilt. An example of this is a patient who was overwhelmed with self-blame for being late for a session. The therapist responded "I'm going to call the police to have you arrested for this!". Such intervention can be felt as supportive, an attempt to diminish the guilt feelings. But there is also the risk that the patient will feel misunderstood or disparaged.

The therapist may use self-deprecating humour to reduce feelings of distance and one-upmanship in the relationship. The humour can convey shared feelings about an external situation. This implicitly involves exposure of some of the therapist's own beliefs and attitudes. This can humanize the therapist and enhance the therapeutic alliance. In making a joke, the therapist is moving out of the "frame" into the real relationship which can be powerfully empathic. This can be a moment of empathic attunement, of meeting, connection and mutual authenticity.

Like all other action alternatives, the expert therapist draws on intuition and System 1 processes. If humour backfires, it can lead to a therapeutic rupture requiring repair and metaprocessing.

Clearly the use of humour should be avoided with patients who have a poorly developed sense of reality or are prone to paranoid misinterpretation.

It is important for the therapist to closely monitor his own feelings, and countertransference as humour may contain hidden aggression. Sharing a joke can involve a collusive irreverence towards a disliked person or institution as a joint expression of anger.

6.6 Action Alternatives: A Provisional Hierarchy

Which interventions when?

Based on a review of the evidence above and the conceptual frameworks used in short-term psychodynamic psychotherapy, I have proposed a provisional hierarchy of action alternatives that can be used to facilitate the therapist's choice of intervention at any point (Fig. 6.1). This must be qualified by recognizing that the evidence available so far is based on linear sequences when in reality interventions occur in repetitive and iterative cycles. Interventions and responses are built on sequences made earlier in the therapeutic session.

Interventions are made to advance the goals of therapy. The optimal intervention may vary depending on the phase of therapy and changes in patient presentation. However the general groupings still apply.

Choices are based on strategies and tactics. Tactics include getting past defences, maintaining the therapeutic alliance and working through emotions.

FIGURE 6.1 Action Alternative Priorities

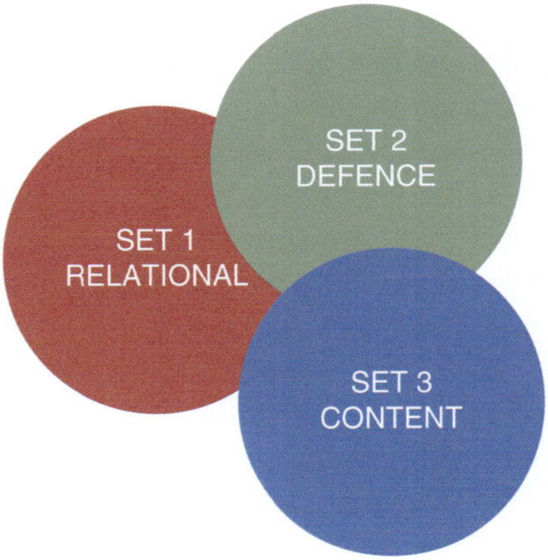

6.6.1 Set 1

Because the research evidence reviewed above points to the therapeutic alliance as one of the strongest predictors of successful therapy, the highest priority choice point action alternatives involve the patient-therapist relationship.

Transference interventions may be regarded as a specific element within this set of interventions.

Within Set 1 the repair of therapeutic ruptures takes priority. If ruptures are not processed, the therapy may be in jeopardy of breakdown. Secondly the working through of ruptures is one of the most powerful therapeutic interventions. It is immediate in the here and now; it involves a corrective emotional experience, a disconfirmation of internal working models and patient expectancies.

Identification and exploration of emotion also belong in priority Set 1, because this is a key component of the therapeutic change process. This comprises helping the patient to identify and express emotion. It is important to "stay with" the emotions in order to process the associated feelings and memories [34].

Emotions can be amplified and deepened by use of metaphor, humour and mental imagery (portrayals).

Dealing with transference is a subset of relational interventions. As mentioned above, too many or too little transference interventions may have a negative impact on treatment outcome. There appears to be an optimal window for this.

Metaprocessing is a higher-order working through of the relationship and leads to a corrective emotional experience and a deeper sense of attachment.

Interventions relating to the relational focus have high priority. These can crystallize the patient's awareness of recurrent patterns of behaviour and the connections to current, past and transference relationships and their associated emotions.

6.6.2 Set 2

- Dealing with defences either by confrontation or bypassing
- Exploring present relationships
- Exploring past relationships
- Clarifying content
- Expressing empathy
- Remaining silent
- Validating

6.6.3 Set 3

- Gathering further information about current or past events
- Providing information
- Psychoeducation

Key Points

- There is evidence to support the importance of the therapeutic alliance, emotion processing and repairing ruptures in achieving good psychotherapy outcomes.
- The therapeutic alliance accounts for about 7.5% of variance in treatment outcome.
- The use of transference interventions may be governed by the "Goldilocks effect". There may be an

optimal "window" for the amount of transference interventions that is dependent on other variables.
- Choice point analysis can be used to select the most effective interventions.
- Selection of action alternatives involves System 2 deliberative thinking.
- Expert therapists are able to make more use of System 1 processes.
- Choice point analysis is an excellent teaching tool.
- Choice points can be recognized by moment-to-moment tracking of emotion and nonverbal cues: facial expression, voice, posture and movement.
- Psychotherapy interventions are not linear but are interactive.
- Psychotherapy is not a closed system. Multiple variables interact in a non-linear fashion making process research complex.

References

1. Tauber L. Choice point analysis-formulation, strategy, intervention, and result in group process therapy and supervision. Int J Group Psychother. 1978;28:163–84.
2. Kahneman D, Tversky A. Choices, values and frames. Am Psychol. 1984;39:341–50.
3. Kahneman D. Thinking fast and slow. Toronto: Anchor Canada; 2013.
4. Metcalfe J, Mischel W. A hot/cool system analysis of delay of gratification: dynamics of willpower. Psychol Rev. 1999;106:3–19.
5. Norman G, Sherbino J, Kelly D, Wood T, Young M, Gaissmaier W, Kreuger S, Monteiro S. The etiology of diagnostic errors: a controlled trial of system 1 versus system 2 reasoning. Acad Med. 2014;89:277–84.
6. Gabbard G. Psychodynamic psychiatry in clinical practice. 5th ed. Washington, DC: APPI; 2014.
7. Gabbard G, Westen D. Rethinking therapeutic action. Int J Psychoanal. 2003;84:823–41.

8. Malan DH. Beyond interpretation: initial evaluation and technique in short-term dynamic psychotherapy. Part I. Int J Short-Term Psychother. 1986;1:59–82.
9. Malan DH. Beyond interpretation: initial evaluation and technique in short-term dynamic psychotherapy. Part II. Int J Short-Term Psychother. 1986;1 83–106.
10. Malan D. The frontier of brief psychotherapy. New York: Plenum; 1976.
11. Davanloo H. Short-term dynamic psychotherapy. New York: Jason Aronson; 1980.
12. Luborsky L. Principles of psychoanalytic psychotherapy: a manual for supportive-expressive treatment. New York: Basic Books; 1984.
13. Fosha D. The transforming power of affect: a model for accelerated change. New York: Basic Books; 2000.
14. McCullogh L, Kuhn N, Andrews S, et al. Treating Affect Phobia a manual for short term dynamic psychotherapy. New York: Guilford press; 2003.
15. Abbass A. Reaching through resistance: advanced psychotherapy techniques. Kansas City: Seven Leaves; 2015.
16. Leichsenring F, Ablon S, Barber JP, et al. Developing a prototype for short-term psychodynamic (supportive-expressive) therapy: an empirical study with the psychotherapy process Q-set. Psychother Res. 2016;26(4):500–10.
17. Horvath AO, Del Re AC, Flückiger C, Symonds D. Alliance in individual psychotherapy. In: Norcross JC, editor. Psychotherapy Relationships that Work. Chapter 2. Oxford University Press; 2011.
18. Diener MJ, Hilsenroth MJ, Weinberger J. Therapist affect focus and patient outcomes in psychodynamic psychotherapy: a meta-analysis. Am J Psychiatry. 2007;164:936–41.
19. Ablon JS, Levy RA, Katzenstein T. Beyond brand names of psychotherapy: identifying empirically supported change processes. Psychother Theory Res Pract Train. 2006;43:216–31.
20. Fisher H, Atzil-Slonim D, Bar-Kalifa E, Rafaeli E, Peri T. Emotional experience and alliance contribute to therapeutic change in psychodynamic therapy. Psychotherapy (Chic). 2016;53(1):105–16.
21. McCarthy KS, Keefe JR, Barber JP. Goldilocks on the couch: moderate levels of psychodynamic and process-experiential technique predict outcome in psychodynamic therapy. Psychother Res. 2016;26:307–17.

22. Marziali EA. Prediction of outcome of brief psychotherapy from therapist interpretive interventions. Arch Gen Psychiatry. 1984;41:301–4.
23. Høglend P, Hersoug AG, Kjell-Petter B, et al. Effects of transference work in the context of therapeutic alliance and quality of object relations. J Consult Clin Psychol. 2011;79(5):697–706.
24. Ulberg R, Amlo S, Høglend P. Manual for transference work scale; a microanalytical tool for therapy process analyses. BMC Psychiatry. 2014;14:291.
25. Safran JD, Muran JC, Samstag LW, Stevens C. Repairing alliance ruptures. In: Norcross JC, editor. Psychotherapy relationships that work. New York: Oxford; 2002. p. 235–55.
26. Samstag LW, Muran JC, Safran JD. Defining and identifying alliance ruptures. In: Charman DP, editor. Core processes in brief psychodynamic psychotherapy: advancing effective practice. London: Lawrence Erlbaum Associates; 2004.
27. Hill C, Knox S. Processing the therapeutic relationship. Psychother Res. 2009;19:13–29.
28. Joyce A, Piper W. Dimensions and predictors of patient response to interpretation. Psychiatry. 1996;59:65–81.
29. Barber J, Crits-Christoph P, Luborsky L. Effects of therapist adherence and competence on patient outcome in brief dynamic therapy. J Consult Clin Psychol. 1996;64(3):619–22.
30. Kubie LS. The destructive potential of humor in psychotherapy. Am J Psychiatry. 1971;127:861–6.
31. Valentine L, Gabbard GO. Can the use of humor in psychotherapy be taught? Acad Psychiatry. 2014;38:75–81.
32. Richman J. The life-saving function of humor with the depressed and suicidal elderly. Gerontologist. 1995;35:271–3.
33. Strick M, Holland RW, van Baaren RB, van Knippenberg A. Those who laugh are defenseless: how humor breaks resistance to influence. J Exp Psychol Appl. 2012;18(2):213–23. https://doi.org/10.1037/a0028534.
34. Prenn N. Mind the gap: AEDP interventions translating attachment theory into clinical practice. J Psychother Integr. 2011;21(3):308–29.

Chapter 7
A Manual for Short-Term Psychodynamic Psychotherapy

7.1 Introduction

The strategic objectives of short-term psychodynamic psychotherapy are to collaborate with the patient to experience and process deep emotions within the framework of a securely attached therapeutic relationship. The goals of STPP are to enhance health and adaptive functioning.

This chapter provides a manualized approach to the conduct of short-term psychodynamic psychotherapy. It details the stages and interventions of STPP [1–15]. The essential and common elements of the various approaches to STPP are synthesized and incorporated into this manual (Chap. 1). Attachment theory (Chap. 2) informs the critically important relational interventions. The identification of action alternatives is derived from choice point analysis (Chap. 6).

Three phases of psychotherapy are presented. Although these are presented sequentially and in a linear fashion in reality, there is an overlap of the tasks and interventions outlined. In practice the boundaries of these phases will shift, and components of the phases will not remain fixed in place. Rather like waves and particles in physics, they will change location and form depending on the dynamics of the observers, in this case the patient and therapist.

The ability to use these approaches depends on extensive clinical practice and supervision. Interventions, as presented

A. Eppel, *Short-Term Psychodynamic Psychotherapy*, https://doi.org/10.1007/978-3-319-74995-2_7

on the written page cannot convey the dynamic and affective nature of the interview process. However this manual can guide students and practitioners in the course of their training and clinical practice.

7.2 The Assessment and Engagement Phase

All of the phases interact and are non-linear (Fig. 7.1). The number of sessions required for assessment and engagement will vary depending on the strength of the patient's defences and attachment style. In some cases, it can be accomplished within the first session; in others it may require three to ten sessions. This will depend on the patient population and the selection criteria being used.

7.2.1 Overall Objectives of the Engagement Phase

Begin to develop a secure base and therapeutic alliance, assess, take the history, evaluate suitability for STPP, orient to treatment process and make a treatment contract.

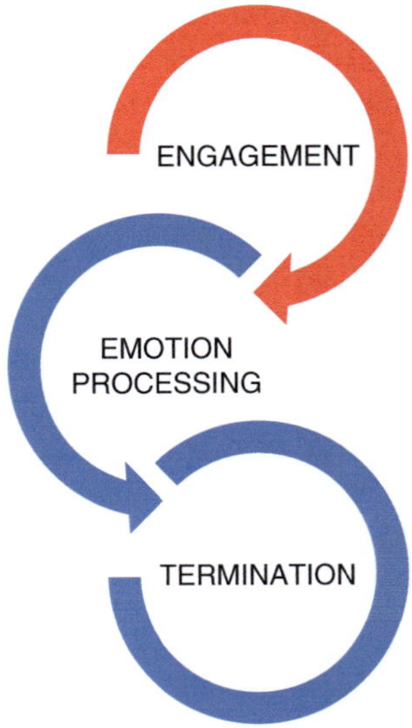

FIGURE 7.1 Engagement

7.2.2 Initial Tasks

Greet patient. Introduce self [16]. Explain roles and the nature of interview. Welcome.

Demonstrate respect and interest. Be nonjudgmental, accepting and authentic in responding to the patient.

Explore the patient's feelings about coming to the interview and their expectations and fears.

If necessary, attend to any disturbing emotions, express empathy and understanding and provide clarification regarding any misconceptions about the process.

7.2.3 Objective: Taking the History

History taking is a dyadic process. What emerges depend on the quality and nature of the interaction between the therapist and patient. The result is a co-constructed narrative. This is why trainees often have the experience of seeing their supervisors elicit a somewhat different history than the one that they had produced.

The components of the history are often determined by the context of the interview and professional and institutional requirements. For beginners history taking often follows a more linear and stilted pattern. For very experienced interviewers, the history emerges fluidly in the process of the dynamic interchange between patient and therapist.

At some point, a general psychiatric history or psychological assessment should be taken. This may have been done prior to the first psychodynamic assessment session.

7.2.4 History Tasks

Presenting problems and history of presenting problems.

Previous psychiatric or psychological treatment.

Prior suicide attempts.

Medical history, substance abuse.

Family history of psychiatric disorder.

Evaluate the mental status and specific risks: suicide, self-harm and aggression.

Explore the patient's problems and the issues that the patient wishes to address with appropriate open-ended questions.

Listen attentively to the patient's opening concerns and history without interrupting or directing patient's response.

Clarify reasons for presenting now, current concerns and symptoms. Explore the onset of the problems, the context in which they occurred and evolution of symptoms.

Clarify patient statements that are unclear or need amplification.

Explore the patient's beliefs and theories about the causes and nature of the problems.

7.2.5 Tasks of Eliciting the Psychodynamic History

In psychodynamic psychotherapy, the history is expanded to include more about early childhood relationships, quality of attachment relationships and patterns of current and past relationships.

Explore the developmental history, family of origin composition.

Explore the nature of the relationship with parents and siblings.

Ask about any specific separations, abuse or trauma.

Explore the attachment style in past and current relationships.

Explore any repetitive relationship patterns and themes.

Explore the patient's view of others. Ask for examples of situations.

Explore the patient's view of himself/herself. Note interaction pattern with therapist.

Explore early attachment relationships.

Identify primary caregivers, i.e. primary attachment relationships.

Ask questions about each of the primary attachment figures (mother, father, siblings, etc.).

Were they loving and affectionate?

During the first session, evaluate the patient's capacity to identify and express emotions. Help patient to express feelings.

Assess patient's ability to reflect.

Evaluate patient's response to a trial interpretation.

7.2.6 Methods

Attend to verbal and non-verbal cues. Track affective changes.

Use open-ended and closed-ended questions to promote the flow of the interview. Avoid jargon and multibarrel questions.

Allow time for patient to reflect before responding.

Use transitional statements or "signposting" when moving to different sections of the interview.

State rationale or context for questions when this may not be obvious to the patient.

Move from general to specific (dilute to concentrate) when exploring sensitive topics.

Demonstrate appropriate non-verbal behaviour: eye contact, facial expression, posture, position and gestures.

Maintain focus on patient's concerns. Avoid distraction by writing notes or using a computer.

Paraphrase or periodically summarize understanding of what the patient has said.

Use gentle commands [17]: "tell me more about that"; "go on"; "stay with that"; and "can you elaborate on that?"

Probe assumptions: "why" and "how" questions designed to challenge patients' presuppositions and unquestioned beliefs.

Challenge the patient's position by asking questions about alternative viewpoints and perspectives, playing both sides of the conflict.

Gentle assumptions [17]: "how many drinks do you usually have on the weekend?"

Use empathic statements: "I sense a lot of pain/sadness. What are you experiencing right now?"

7.2.6.1 Attachment-Based Questions

These questions elicit information about early attachment relationships and the experience of attachment and separation in adulthood. These provide qualitative information and are not scored (Table 7.1). These questions can be used separately for each of the patient's primary attachment figures.

TABLE 7.1 Attachment-based questions

Part one: childhood		
When I was a child, my mother/father/primary caregiver:	Mostly yes	Mostly no
Was loving		
Was affectionate		
Was distant		
Was critical		
Used physical punishment		
Was away a lot		
Left me alone a lot		
Made me feel safe		
Made me feel unsafe		
Mistreated me		
Hugged me a lot		
Spent time with me		
Abused me		
Cuddled me		
Showed affection		
When I was upset, my mother comforted me		
When I was hurt or ill, my mother comforted me		
Was not interested in me		
Threatened to leave me when I misbehaved		

TABLE 7.1 (continued)

Part two: separation

When I first went to school, I was happy	Mostly yes	Mostly no
I looked forward to going to school		
I was fearful and anxious about going to school		
I was very happy when I moved out of my parents' home		
I was anxious and fearful when I first lived on my own		
I am not able to live alone because I get lonely		
I like to travel		
I prefer to stay home		

Part three: adult relationships

When I am dating, I worry all the time that my boyfriend/girlfriend will leave me	Mostly yes	Mostly no
I am possessive of my boyfriend/girlfriend		
I need to phone or text my boyfriend/girlfriend many times a day to make sure he/she still loves me		
I am afraid of getting close to others		
Needing someone makes me feel weak		
I am able to share my private feelings with people close to me		
I quickly break up relationships when I sense my boyfriend/girlfriend no longer loves me		
I am sensitive to rejection		
I easily feel abandoned		
I take care of other people so that they won't leave me		
I prefer to rely on myself not on other people		

7.3 The Relational Focus

The relational focus is a unique component of short-term dynamic psychotherapies. Michael Balint first described this concept which he called "focal psychotherapy" [1, 2] Lester Luborsky [8] developed a similar concept known as the core conflictual relationship theme which gained wide acceptance [10].

The identification of a relational focus or core theme is very important for the practice of short-term psychodynamic psychotherapies. It helps to limit the scope of the therapy which in turn reduces the length of therapy. It allows the patient to develop a more coherent narrative and view of himself. The relational focus provides insight into relational patterns and difficulties. It serves as a reference point for interpretations throughout the course of the therapy. Sharing the relational focus with the patient in written as well as verbal form enhances the collaborative aspects of the therapeutic alliance.

During the course of early childhood the developing brain begins to build up a picture of the external environment. The external environment includes the physical as well as the social environments. The brain constructs a map of the external environment in order to enhance survival. The organism needs to predict what it may encounter in the external world.

In a similar fashion, the child develops internal models both of himself and of other humans in his environment. Early relationships with attachment figures lead to the formation of an internal working model (Chap. 2). In object relations language, this is called internalized self and object representations. These internalized models form a template for all subsequent relationships (Fig. 7.2).

The models are referred to as templates, schemas and self-object representations depending on the particular theoretical language one uses.

The internal working models are shaped by the multiple interactions the child has with the physical environment and with other people. The first 3–5 years of life are critical for the development of these templates.

Clearly these templates will be influenced mostly by the primary attachment figures within the child's life.

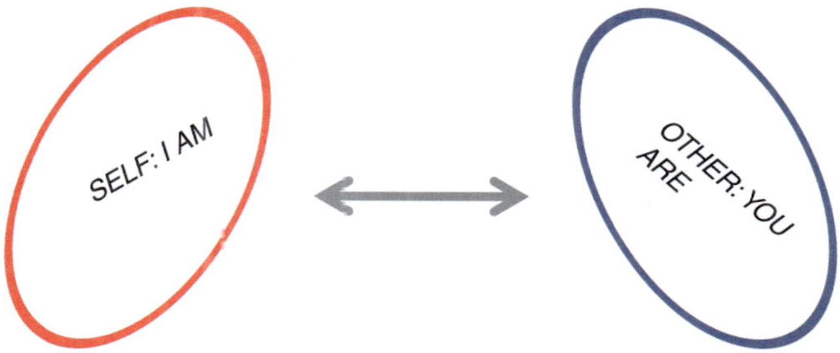

FIGURE 7.2 The self-other relational focus

An internal working model has two components: a sense, feeling and image of our self and a sense, feeling and image of other people. These two components of the model are joined and are linked by various emotions.

The self-other models comprise part of conscious awareness of ourselves but also nonconscious and implicit information (Chap. 3).

These repetitive patterns are evident in current relationships, past relationships and the relationship with the therapist.

The relational focus is the outward manifestation of the internal model. It is made up of the patient's view of himself and his expectations and views of others (Table 7.2). The patient may have some awareness of his view of himself and of others but much of this is implicit and manifests unconsciously.

7.3.1 *Identifying the Relational Focus*

This is derived from the early interviews based on information about the patient's early and current relationships, his/her attachment style and most validly from the nature of the interaction between the patient and the therapist. Various questionnaires as mentioned in Sect. 7.1 can be used to complement or validate the clinical assessment.

How does the patient experience himself in relationship to others? What are his implicit expectations about how others will treat him?

Table 7.2 The relational focus

Self: I am	Other: you are
Unworthy/unlovable/alone	Abandoning
Submissive/dependent/passive	Dominating
Incompetent/weak/stupid	Powerful
Blameworthy	Blaming
Shameful	Shaming
Undesirable	Rejecting/critical
Not good enough/defective	Devaluing
Helpless/vulnerable	Controlling
Untrusting	Abusive
Invisible	Dismissive
A failure	Humiliating
Deserving of punishment	Critical

Any of the self representations in the left hand column can be paired with any of the other person representations in the right hand column

How does the patient view others? How do they perceive him?

A detailed review of precipitating events or major interpersonal ruptures can help identify core themes. The key relationship dynamics may be evident. The precipitating event may contain a crystallization of the core theme and lead to identification of a primary focus.

The engagement phase continues over one to three sessions. During this period, the therapeutic alliance is fostered by promoting a secure attachment to the therapist.

This is achieved by means of attunement to the patient's feelings and the expression of genuine empathy and validation.

The provisional relational focus should be reviewed with the patient, and a written description of this should be given to the patient. As therapy proceeds, the focus may become more defined and specific leading to more accurate interventions.

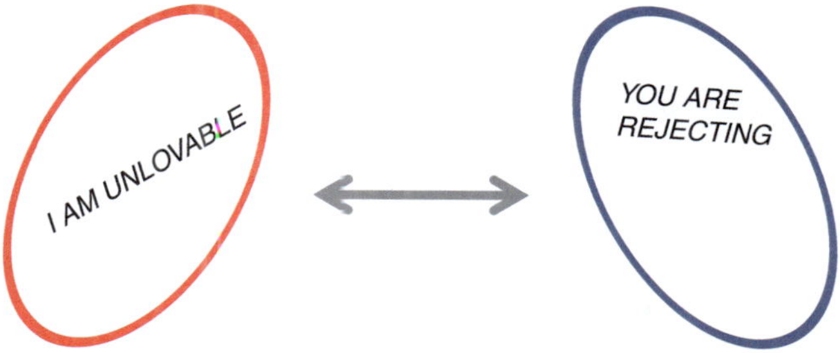

FIGURE 7.3 Relational focus example

A verbal treatment contract should be negotiated and an orientation given to the process of therapy and contingencies. The treatment contract can specify a number of sessions, e.g. 6, 12, 16, 20 or 40, or be based on a specific termination date. In the latter case, missed sessions cannot be made up (Fig. 7.3).

7.4 Suitability for STPP

There are some general guidelines that can be used to assess whether the patient will benefit from STPP and whether they will be able to successfully engage in it. Even with guidelines, there are many therapist factors that influence the decision to engage a patient in treatment. The question of who can benefit from STPP is an empirical one. However because of the limitations of our diagnostic systems and variations in practice, it is not possible to be definitive. The status of research does not provide an answer to the ultimate question of "which patients do best with which form of psychotherapy and with which type of therapist?" The following guidelines are based on a synthesis of current practice, literature and experience:

- A capacity to identify and reflect on emotions
- An interest in reflecting on what is happening in his/her life as opposed to primarily seeking symptom relief from practical strategies

- The patient is curious about his/her role in his/her difficulties
- Experiencing some distress
- Motivated to make changes
- Has at least one significant relationship
- Has a capacity to form an alliance with the therapist
- The patient displays a positive response to the therapist's attempts to understand him/her
- Recurring problematic patterns in interpersonal relationships
- Problems with self-concept
- Maladaptive defences

7.4.1 Attachment Style

This is reflected in the patient's narrative style (Chap. 2). If the patient's account is poorly organized and lacks coherence, the patient may have a disorganized attachment style. This can be further evaluated during the assessment. Patients with disorganized attachment are not likely to benefit from STPP.

Patients with secure attachment as reflected in their ability to have successful relationships are excellent candidates for STPP.

For the other categories of attachment, dismissing, avoidant and fearful, suitability for STPP will depend on the intensity of these attachment characteristics. Some of these patients will require longer-term psychotherapy.

7.4.2 Diagnostic Considerations

A specific diagnosis is not a necessary or sufficient factor for suitability for STPP. Patient characteristics such as intensity of symptoms and their impact on their ability to participate in psychotherapy are more important than phenomenological diagnosis. More often than not, patients have multiple diagnoses which is an artefact of our classification systems. This will also depend on the setting in which patients are seen.

Patients with diagnoses of depression, generalized anxiety disorder, social anxiety disorder, panic disorder, post-traumatic stress disorder and trauma-related problems that do not meet diagnostic threshold for PTSD are suitable for STPP.

Patients with moderate or severe obsessive compulsive disorder do not appear to benefit from STPP. Cognitive behaviour therapy can be effective.

Patients with grief, relationship conflicts and personality disorder should be considered for STPP.

Patients with obsessive-compulsive personality disorder, dependent personality and avoidant personality should also be considered.

Patients with borderline traits may be considered depending on severity. Patients with high levels of emotional dysregulation, frequent self-harm or suicide attempts may require alternate forms of psychotherapy such as dialectical behaviour therapy or transference-focused psychotherapy.

Patients with bipolar disorder who are stable on medications are suitable for STPP.

Treatment with psychotropic medications is not a contraindication for STPP.

The patient's social and occupational environment, should be relatively stable. If there is ongoing trauma or environmental crises, it will not be possible to focus on the tasks of therapy. Periodic crises will derail the therapy focus. Therapy may have to be switched to a supportive crisis intervention mode.

Patients who have ongoing psychosis or organic cognitive impairments are unable to participate in STPP.

Patients with high levels of antisocial, narcissistic, schizoid and schizotypal traits are not suitable for STPP.

7.4.3 Contract and Orientation

Towards the end of the first session, ask the patient to express his/her goals for the therapy.

Explain the treatment process.

Emphasize the patient's active role which will be necessary if the treatment is to be successful. Explain the therapist's role.

"Your role is to say what you need to say about yourself about events and about how you feel in the treatment. I will listen and respond whenever it is likely to be helpful".

Give the patient an opportunity to express any doubts about the usefulness of the treatment.

Explore the patient's ambivalence about changing versus remaining the same. Explore both sides of the ambivalence.

Discuss the logistics and practical arrangements for the treatment including duration and frequency of sessions.

Discuss arrangements for missed or cancelled sessions.

Discuss number of sessions or length of treatment and termination date.

Negotiate one of two methods for contracting termination:

- A fixed number of sessions between 8 and 40 sessions. In this method, missed or cancelled sessions may be made up.
- A fixed date ending. In this method therapy is ended on a pre-agreed date even if some sessions have been missed by patient.

In either case, there should be a "hard" termination, i.e. therapy is not extended as the termination process is an intrinsic part of the therapeutic effect.

Explore the patient's feelings about time limits: e.g. the proposal to meet for 12 sessions may be interpreted as "I can only tolerate you for 12 sessions" or "you are not deserving of longer treatment".

Clarify these feelings at the beginning of therapy emphasizing the therapeutic reasons for the time limit.

7.4.4 Orientation to Therapy: A Sample Narrative

"At today's meeting I want to talk with you about how this therapy works and how it is done.

The purpose of this therapy is to help you overcome your difficulties. This form of therapy has been successfully used for the treatment of many types of problems such as depression, general anxiety, panic, social anxiety, trauma, interpersonal difficulties, dealing with physical illness, grief, loss, problems in relationships.

This form of therapy is focused on helping you to get in touch and to express feelings that have been buried or blocked from your awareness. These feelings are connected with unresolved issues in your life that affect your view of your self and your view of other people. These unresolved issues can interfere with your relationships, mood and levels of anxiety resulting in problems in your life and clinical symptoms.

Emotions are central to all that we do. Emotions prepare us for dealing with our environment. The emotion of fear prepares us to deal with danger. The emotion of sadness helps us deal with separation and loss. The emotion of joy allows us to explore and engage with others. The emotion of love connects us with others. The emotion of anger allows us to deal with threats to our integrity.

All of us exhibit certain patterns in our close relationships. These patterns are based on our early relationships and early environment. In particular they are influenced by our early attachment relationships. Attachment is the emotional bond between the infant and its mother. During the child's development there may be several different people that play a primary role as an attachment figure. Frequently this is the mother or father but can be a grandparent, older sibling or other caregiver. The people with whom the infant has the most contact are known as the primary attachment figures. If the primary attachment figures respond to our needs as infants for soothing, affection, warmth and food we will grow up with a positive sense of ourselves and of the world around us. If on the other hand the quality of the attachment relationships is inconsistent, this will lead to insecurities in our view of ourselves and the world. Finally if we have been exposed to physical, sexual or emotional abuse this will have a profound impact on our self-image and our views of other people.

Our early attachment relationships form the prototype for future relationships. In a sense we take in to ourselves a template of common relationship patterns. These templates are known as internal working models and are based on the myriad of relationships and interactions we have in early childhood. The first 3–5 years of life are especially critical for laying down some of the basic components of the templates.

These templates shape our expectations and perceptions when we enter into new relationships; they shape our perceptions of the other person's response to us.

These relationship templates can lead to maladaptive patterns of relating resulting in repeated difficulties in close and intimate relationships. These maladaptive patterns often lie at the basis of the problems that bring you into therapy.

In the therapy I will be helping you identify these patterns and the impact they have on your relationships and your emotions.

These patterns reoccur in your current close relationships, in your past relationships but also in your relationship with me the therapist. This can be difficult to talk about in therapy but is an essential part of the treatment process.

How Is Therapy Done?

Sessions will be held once or twice a week. We will decide in advance the number of sessions, e.g. 8, 16, 24, depending on the nature of your problems. Once the length of treatment is agreed upon by you and me, this is fixed as it is important to have a firm ending in order to get the full benefit of the treatment.

Each session will last for approximately 50 min.

You and I are expected to arrive on time and will commit to that.

If for any reason you have to cancel the session, it would be appreciated if you could do that as soon as possible. If however you frequently miss sessions, this will interfere with the flow of the therapy, and it may not be possible to continue. Therapy may have to be ended although could be reconsidered in the future.

This type of therapy is generally not about giving advice. The problems that you are facing cannot be solved by simple advice. However by means of clarification and understanding your own inner feelings and wishes, you will be better able to make your own choices and decisions. It is never a case of the therapist knows best. Rather you and I work together grappling with the issues to reach clarity and emotional resolution.

This therapy differs from other approaches such as cognitive behaviour therapy. The primary focus in cognitive therapy is on thinking patterns and exposure to feared situations. In depression and anxiety, distorted patterns of thinking can be identified, e.g. catastrophizing, mind-reading and all or nothing thinking. In dynamic psychotherapy the focus is on emotional processing although distorted thinking may also be challenged. It may be conceptualized differently as a form of defence.

Concurrent Therapies

Prior to starting therapy, you will have had a full psychological or psychiatric evaluation to ensure that this form of therapy is suitable for you. It may be necessary to attend to physical health problems prior to commencing therapy. If so you will be advised to see your family physician or nurse practitioner.

In the event that you are being prescribed psychotropic medications, a decision will need to be made whether your therapist or family physician will be in charge of this part of your treatment. This will of course depend on whether or not your therapist has prescribing privileges. This will vary from jurisdiction to jurisdiction.

It is generally recommended that you not engage in different forms of psychotherapy concurrently with our therapy. It may be appropriate following completion of our therapy for you to engage in other forms of therapy.

How Are Sessions Conducted?

You as the patient have the role of starting off each session. You are free to speak about whatever is on your mind. Often patients at the beginning of therapy worry that they won't have anything to say and try to plan or rehearse for the next session. This is neither required nor beneficial. Very quickly you will find that you have no difficulty talking about things that are on your mind. My job will be to help you clarify what is important to the treatment, to help you identify, express and experience important emotions and to begin to understand how relationship patterns affect your moods and relationships.

I will frequently point out evidence of emotions and help you focus on these emotions and give them expression. Because this is often difficult, you may find that you have habitual ways of deflecting or diverting from painful emotions. It is my job to keep you on target so that we can get to the core feelings. This may involve me challenging some of your ways of defending yourself emotionally.

In the course of therapy, you may develop strong positive or negative feelings towards me. This is expected and indeed is a central part of the treatment process. These feelings will often parallel components of your relationship patterns. The ability of us to explore and discuss these feelings and reflect on them is a very important part of treatment.

Sometimes you may feel that you do want to come to a session. Maybe you feel angry towards me or feel embarrassed or anxious about something you said. It is most important at these times that you do in fact come to the session to discuss these very feelings. These kinds of feelings are often related to the main issues that you are dealing with and discussing them with me can be extremely helpful for your progress.

I will give you some assessment forms to fill out at the beginning of treatment. This is to provide more detail about the nature and severity of your problems.

At the end of treatment, you will complete some of the same measures to see what has changed for the better. There are also some other outcome measures that we will discuss to evaluate the effects of the treatment.

The last phase of treatment is called termination. This word is powerful and somewhat ominous. Nevertheless it is apt because termination is a very powerful and important step in the whole process of therapy. Something is ending and that can create the same types of feelings that one experiences after a loss or a death of someone close. These are universal feelings and reflecting upon them is very helpful for the therapy. In the words of the old French poem 'Partir c'est mourir un peu' – leaving is to die a little. Loss is painful but when processed can enhance resilience. I will focus on termination issues in approximately the last third of our sessions. During this time many of the same issues may become intensified due to the approaching end of treatment.

7.5 The Emotion Processing and Thematic Phase

This is often described as the middle phase of therapy but the therapy may shift back and forth (Fig. 7.4).

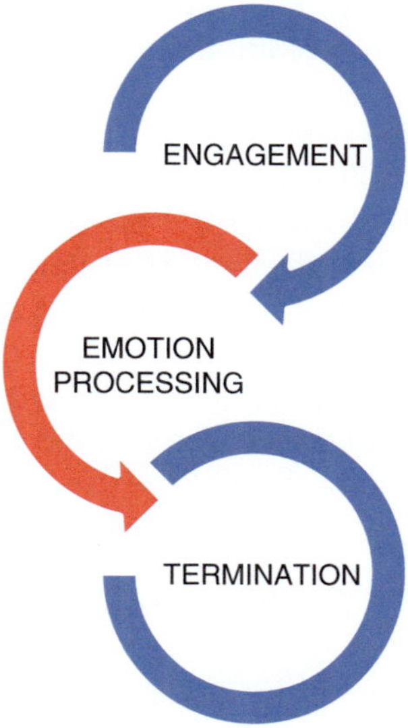

FIGURE 7.4 The emotion processing phase

TABLE 7.3 Defences

Group I	**Group II**	**Group III**
Adaptive or maladaptive	**Maladaptive**	**Highly adaptive**
Repression	Projection	Altruism
Displacement	Acting out	Sublimation
Rationalization	Dissociation	Humour
Intellectualization	Splitting	
Reaction formation	Idealization	
Isolation of affect	Somatization	

Sessions 4 to 16.

Tactically all forms of psychodynamic psychotherapy have a similar approach which is to get past psychological defences to reach core feelings.

Core feelings are linked to the patient's internal working models. This manifests in the patient's recurrent interpersonal patterns which are related to the presenting problems and difficulties in the patient's life.

It is the experience and processing of these often unconscious emotions that are more powerfully therapeutic than interpretation and insight.

To get to these deep emotions, it is necessary to get past the patient's defences.

Davanloo refers to this as "unlocking the unconscious". Fosha describes the parallel process as "dropping down" to core affect and core state.

It is important to be familiar with the range and types of defences (Table 7.3).

The use of the two triangles, dealing with transference and countertransference and making interpretations, are also central to this phase.

7.5.1 Tactical Defences

The term "tactical defences" was coined by Davanloo [4, 5] in contradistinction to the traditional defences described by Sigmund Freud and Anna Freud. These defences are among the most commonly observed in psychotherapy

TABLE 7.4 Tactical defences

Vagueness	Laughing and smiling	Not remembering
Talking to avoid feelings	Blaming	Passive compliance
Alterations in rate of speech	Avoiding eye contact	Argumentativeness
Humour and sarcasm	Overgeneralization	Rumination and repetition
Use of jargon	Seductiveness	Shallow weepiness
Helplessness	Avoidant posture	Intimidation

(Table 7.4). They act to distance the patient from his feelings and to disqualify them. Tactical defences also can divert the therapist from focusing on important material. Davanloo introduced the technique of challenging these firmly but supportively. It is the defences that are challenged not the patient.

7.5.2 *Using the Triangle of Defence and the Triangle of the Person*

Major objectives of the middle phase are to get past defences in order to reach core feelings (in this context the words "emotions", "affects" and "feelings" are often used interchangeably reflecting the lack of agreement on the definitions of these terms. See Chap. 3).

The triangle of defence provides an excellent tool to achieve these objectives (Chap. 1).

At any moment in a session, the patient may be experiencing distress in the form of anxiety, guilt or shame, or these feelings may be pushed out of awareness by the operation of defences. These two modes are represented on the corners of the triangle. Emotion is located at the bottom of the triangle. This represents deep visceral emotion such as sadness, anger, joy, grief and rage (See Chap. 1) (Fig. 7.5).

The objective is to "get to the bottom of the triangle", i.e. to the expression of emotion.

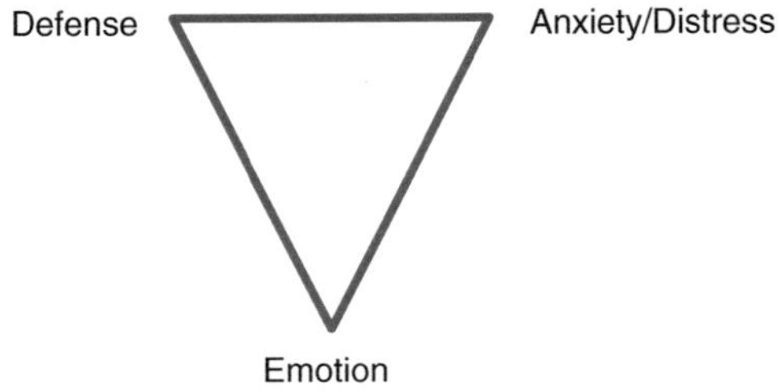

FIGURE 7.5 Triangle of conflict

7.5.2.1 Intervention Tasks

The interventions described here are based largely on the work of Diana Fosha, Natasha Prenn and David Malan [5, 9, 17].

Continuously track verbal and non-verbal signals.

Observe defensive patterns.

Observe and challenge tactical defences.

Point out defensive patterns. Make explicit the benefits and costs of the defences [9].

Defences have protected you from terrible pain but led to maladaptive relationships and symptoms.

Bypass or confront defences.

Explore the feelings behind defences: fear, anger, grief-sadness, joy, sexuality and attachment/love.

Identify and stay with core emotions like sadness, aloneness, grief, anger, rage and joy:

"How did you feel?"

"How do you feel now...talking about it?"

Attenuate pathogenic emotions of guilt, shame, aloneness and hopelessness by means of empathy, acceptance and reframing.

Regulate level of anxiety and emotional arousal by varying use of supportive and emotion-eliciting interventions.

Identify bodily signs of feeling: *where in your body do you feel it?*

Describe what it feels like

.......stay with the feeling.

Get to the bottom of the triangle.

Encourage full expression of emotions and associated memories.

Enhance the alliance. Convey acceptance, empathy and validation.

Help reshape/reframe the perceptions and meanings attached to emotionally charged memories.

Experiential language [17]:

- Use small words.
- Use short statements or questions one at a time.
- Slow down and wait.
- Be specific or be vague. Be specific to challenge tactical defences and to clarify ambiguity.

Be vague by using incomplete sentences to avoid premature closure or conclusions:

'Let's slow this down'; 'let's take a breath here'; 'we have time'; 'let's pause

here'; 'let's go back'; 'let's stay here'; 'let's stay with this';

Ask permission 'can we...?' [17]

Use short clear words. The interventions should be concise and not long-winded. Statements are often more effective than questions. Use simple language. Repeat interventions for emphasis.

Use visual imagery (portrayals) and metaphor to amplify experience of emotion.

Explore positive emotions such as joy and pride as well as painful emotions: anger, sadness, grief and disgust.

Diana Fosha states that the unit of intervention is not the therapist's comment but the therapist's comment and the patient's response. What matters is the patient's experience of the intervention and his/her subsequent response. The therapist can make an empathic intervention, but it is important to explore whether or not the patient experiences it as empathic [9].

Metaprocess the experience of the therapeutic relationship: *How does it feel to tell me about this? What did it feel like for you when I said you are too hard on yourself?*

How did you feel when I was late?

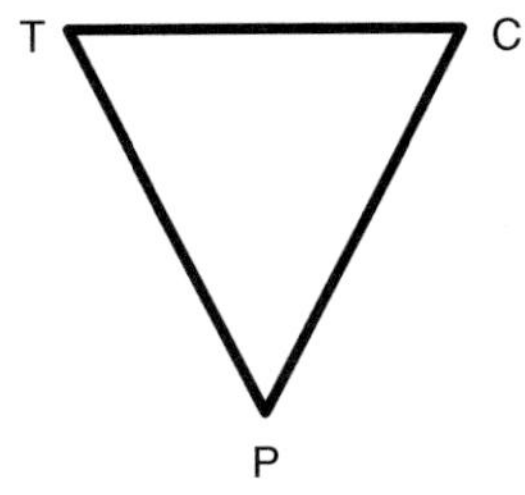

FIGURE 7.6 Triangle of the person. T transference relationship, C current relationship patterns, P past relationship patterns

7.5.2.2 Transference: Triangle of the Person

The relational focus manifests in all of the patient's relationships.

It appears in current relationships with family, spouses, friends, bosses, etc. It is evident in the childhood relationships with the primary attachment figures. It also becomes apparent in the relationship with the therapist, i.e. in the transference relationship.

The therapist can gain insight into the focal pattern by becoming aware of his own emotional responses to the patient. His real reaction and countertransference responses provide useful information and understanding on what is happening in the therapeutic relationship.

The triangle of the person can be used to point out to the patient how the relational focus is linked to his early relationships and is evident in his current relationships and his relationship with the therapist (Fig. 7.6).

7.6 The Formulation

After the first two to three sessions, a provisional formulation can be developed. The formulation consists of understanding the relational focus, the associated emotions, the patient's defences and the impact of all this on his/her behaviour, symptoms and psychological functioning.

The tentative formulation should be shared with the patient in the session so that the patient can contribute to it and test the goodness of fit. As part of this therapy protocol, the patient should be given a written copy of the formulation.

An example of a hypothetical case vignette is presented, and the formulation is demonstrated in Table 7.3.

Case Vignette 7.1

Veronica is a 37-year-old single woman who has depression and social anxiety. She describes her parents as having been emotionally detached showing little overt affection. At the same time, they tended to be critical. They disapproved of her choice of career in healthcare. She could never do enough to please them. She has given up on close relationships as she always feels taken advantage of. At work she finds that she is always staying late. When asked to do extra work or coverage is needed, she is the one that volunteers. She is feeling burnt out (Tables 7.2 and 7.5).

In therapy Veronica would be made aware of the relational focus: how repeatedly in close relationships both in the past and in the present she is self-sacrificing. Her nonconscious expectation is that she will be dismissed or criticized. One could predict that in her relationship with the therapist, this relational theme will emerge. She may feel that the therapist is uncaring and dismissive despite her efforts to be a model patient.

TABLE 7.5 Relational focus written formulation example

Veronica's view of herself	Unworthy, unlovable
View of others	Critical, dismissive
Effects on behaviour	Self-sacrificing, needing to please
Associated emotions	Resentment, unexpressed, anger, depression
Defences	Reaction formation, repression

7.7 Choice Point Analysis and Action Alternatives in the Therapeutic Phase

At any instant during a therapy session, the therapist has multiple action alternatives to choose from. Lewis Tauber developed a system which he called "choice point analysis" for use in supervising trainee group therapists [18] (Chap. 6). There are points during the psychotherapeutic session which call for an intervention or response by the therapist. This could be signalled by changes in emotion, speech quality, posture and eye contact. The expression of defences may also need to be addressed. Silence, avoidance, expression of anger or negative comments towards the therapist all require exploration.

Many of these action choices become intuitive for experienced therapists, but self-reflection and self-monitoring need to be exercised. Interventions must be considered in the light of therapeutic goals and tactics. Interventions are made to advance the goals of therapy.

In order to guide the therapy process, I have attempted to group action alternatives into three sets in order of priority. This is based on my review of the process research literature examining the effectiveness of different interventions on treatment outcome (Chap. 6). These action alternatives are particularly useful for the training and supervision of students but are also relevant to experienced therapists (Chap. 9).

7.7.1 A Provisional Hierarchy of Action Alternatives

I have grouped the principal action alternatives in three sets in order of priority (Fig. 7.7).

7.7.2 Choice Point Action Alternatives Set One: Relational

These consist of actions pertaining to the development and maintenance of the therapeutic alliance. Because the

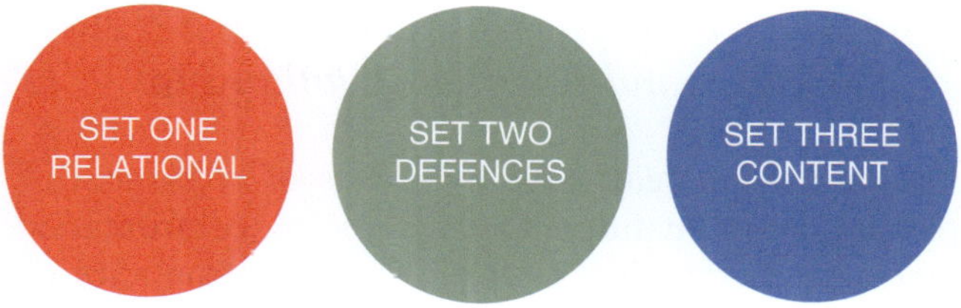

FIGURE 7.7 Choice point actions

therapeutic alliance is one of the strongest predictors of successful psychotherapy, interventions of this nature are given the highest priority. These action alternatives relate to the patient therapist relationship and are referred to as "relational interventions" [9]. Relational interventions indicate collaboration: *I am here to help, you are not alone, and we are in this together.* The deliberate use of the word "we" highlights the attachment relationship in the moment [9].

Set one action alternatives include the following:

Maintaining the therapeutic alliance.

Acknowledging and repairing therapeutic ruptures including transference issues.

Metaprocessing.

Working with the relational focus.

Priority is also given to interventions that facilitate the expression and experience of emotion.

Emotion-focused strategies include facilitating genuine expression of core emotions, encouragement to stay with and tolerate deepening of emotional experience.

Amplifying emotion experience by focusing on the bodily experience of emotion and the use of visual imagery such as portrayals.

Portrayals involve imagining particular events or scenarios and describing the feelings experienced as if the events were occurring in the present moment. This technique can induce rapid access to intense emotion that is connected it to particular memories.

7.7.3 Choice Point Action Alternatives Set Two: Defences and External Relationships

Defences can be dealt with by means of confrontation or bypassing. A premature or too vigorous confrontation of defences can lead to their intensification. Confrontation of the defences as they manifest in the transference is a key strategy in Davanloo's intensive short-term dynamic psychotherapy. However this is carefully guided by monitoring the nature of the transference and the patient's level of anxiety [13, 14].

Again Diana Fosha has demonstrated masterful technique in her approach to bypassing or "melting" defences. By means of deep attunement to the patient, genuine empathy and the use of specific forms of self-disclosure, the patient is able to relinquish defences and access emotions.

Provoking curiosity can be used to arouse the patient's interest in examining his/her defences:

It is interesting that every time I ask you how you are feeling you start to talk about your recent vacation. I noticed that when we get close to something painful you make a joke. I wonder why that might be?

For patients with secure attachment, tactical defences can be directly challenged. This is a major technical innovation developed by Davanloo. It involves pointing out that the defence works against the patient's best interests: *when we talk about your mother's death, you become vague and ramble on. How does this help you come to terms with your feelings?*

Action two alternatives also include exploring present relationships and past relationships. These relationships do not have the same priority as the therapeutic relationship and the transference.

7.7.4 Choice Point Action Alternatives Set Three: Content

These actions relate more to content than to process. At times during therapy, it is necessary to go back to get more history or to clarify information or events. Discrepancies in reported information may need to be clarified or explored.

The use of silence may be appropriate at certain points in a session. This has been referred to as "being with" the patient rather than "doing with."

Providing information and psychoeducation is included in set three. This should be evaluated to ensure that this is not diversionary intellectualization.

7.8 Termination

Termination is difficult for patients but also difficult for the therapist and perhaps particularly so for beginning therapists and supervisees. Termination is always lurking in the background throughout all phases (Fig. 7.8).

The response to termination will depend on how successful the therapy has been. In long-term psychotherapy, therapy is continued until a mutually agreed termination point. Short-term psychodynamic psychotherapy is deliberately different.

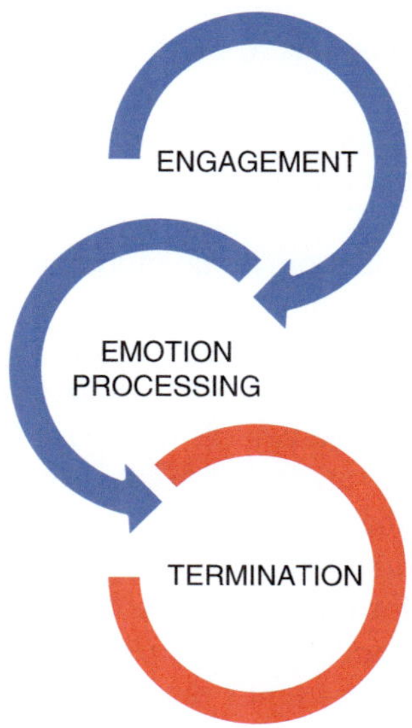

FIGURE 7.8 The termination phase

A hard termination is preferred which can be a fixed number of sessions or specific termination date. This hard termination is a therapeutic strategy and not just one of maximizing efficiency and resources.

James Mann emphasized the benefits of a fixed termination which in fact leads to the acceleration of the therapeutic process. This is somewhat analogous to Parkinson's law. Parkinson was a British civil servant who wrote that "Work expands so as to fill the time available for its completion" [19]. The so-called Stock-Sanford corollary of this states that "if you wait until the last minute, it only takes a minute to do". While these sayings represent folklore surprisingly, they mirror the experience of short- and long-term psychotherapy.

A criticism of long-term psychotherapy is its tendency to linger and to lose focus. In Freud's felicitous phrase, this was "analysis interminable" [20]. Freud wrote this paper in 1937 about a patient for whom he had felt that progress had stopped. Freud believed that his patient felt comfortable in the current situation and did not have any wish to take any step which would bring him nearer to the end of treatment. Freud resorted to the "heroic measure" of fixing a time limit for the analysis. He informed the patient that "the coming year was to be the last one of our treatment, no matter what he achieved in the time still left to him". Freud says that the patient's resistances shrank in that much was accomplished in the last months of treatment.

Termination is obviously most difficult when themes of rejection or abandonment are important or constitute the relational focus. In those cases, termination should be addressed much earlier in the therapy, while there is at least a third of sessions remaining.

The patient may wish to avoid facing the prospect of termination and display formal and tactical defences: intellectualization, isolation of feeling, diversion, overinclusiveness and distraction. It is therefore important that the therapist throughout the course of therapy frequently sets marker points as to the number of remaining sessions and explores the patient's reactions to these reminders along the way.

The therapist may also unconsciously wish to avoid facing termination. This may be due to countertransferential issues relating to the therapist's own experiences with separation and loss. The therapist may be unaware of his/her own sadness at the prospect of termination.

For beginning therapists, the feeling that termination is going to be painful for the patient may lead to discomfort or feelings of guilt. The therapist may feel that the patient needs more time and that they have not completed the job.

This is evident in supervision when the supervisee is reminded that it is time to address termination issues yet fails to do so in subsequent sessions. Many supervisees will readily volunteer that they have difficulty with termination, and the conscious barriers to this can be discussed during supervision.

Where therapy has not been effective in whole or in part, termination may be contentious. Either party may wish that the therapy could continue. The patient may express disappointment and anger that the promised results have not been attained. The patient may attempt to pressure the therapist to extend the length of therapy despite the therapeutic contract outlining a hard termination. This pressure may go as far as the patient threatening to complain to the therapist's supervisor or manager. An attempt to work through these emotions in the context of the relational focus may be helpful. Freud described the setting of a time limit as a "blackmailing device". He felt that this technique could not be fully effective because a large amount of the material will be suppressed under the pressure of the time limit.

Freud did make the important point that once a time limit has been set, the therapist cannot retract it; "otherwise the patient would lose all faith in him". It should be noted though that Freud's patient referred to above, required several further months of treatment with him. After he had returned from the war as a refugee, he needed intermittent treatment over subsequent years.

We can now say that this issue is one that is subject to empirical testing. In any case at the time of termination, the patient may feel that many issues or symptoms are not fully resolved. If that is the case, considerations of alternative forms of therapy and referral to these are quite appropriate.

At the same time, the expression of disappointment or criticism of the therapist in the context of termination may represent the relational theme in the transference. It may reflect the expression of anger directed towards the therapist for abandoning him/her. This of course needs to be processed and worked through and may have an important positive therapeutic impact.

Conversely the patient may express thankfulness and positive regard towards the therapist which may in fact be a defensive cover for underlying feelings of anger or sadness at the ending of therapy. Regardless of the firm contract, the patient may challenge the therapist insisting that it must be possible to modify the contract. This anger may be displaced onto institutional policies.

Patients may of course terminate therapy prematurely. This action has multiple meanings understandable in the context of the selected relational focus. For those with avoidant attachment style, dropping out of treatment may represent a pre-emptive strike to forestall the experience of rejection. In other cases, it may be an attempt to frustrate the therapist or to demonstrate the therapist's ineffectiveness and incompetence.

An attempt should therefore be made to reengage the patient in order to explore these themes and work them through. This can be done by telephoning the patient or sending a letter or email. A letter may be preferable as it allows the sender and the receiver more time to contemplate the message and the response. It should be pointed out in the letter that the patient's desire to terminate therapy early is an important treatment issue and that exploring this can have immense therapeutic value.

The question arises as to whether there should be any a post-termination follow-up. The idea that treatment can be restarted in the future may undermine the value of the hard termination contract. An agreement to undertake an outcome follow-up session after 1 year can be built into the initial contract with the understanding that therapy would not be restarted regardless of the patient's status. Referrals to other treatment can be recommended. The reason for this is that if therapy is reinitiated or extended at any point, then there is no possibility of effecting proper termination.

Focus on termination should begin when there are about one third of the sessions remaining.

Discussion of termination should begin sooner when there are issues relating to abandonment, rejection or separation.

7.8.1 Termination Tasks

Norcross and colleagues surveyed 65 psychotherapists practising across five different psychotherapy models to determine which interventions were used during the termination process [21]. Surprisingly there was a very high agreement across the five psychotherapy orientations about these interventions. The experts worked from an 80-item survey to reach consensus. Eighteen of these items were endorsed by 80 to 89% of the experts, and 13 interventions were endorsed by 70–79%. The following termination tasks are based on these findings which had a high level of consensus:

- Explore the patient's feelings of loss.
- Anticipate both positive and negative reactions in therapist.
- Beware of countertransference.
- Process patient's feelings about ending the therapeutic relationship.
- Anticipate both positive and negative reactions from the patient.
- Discuss patient's future functioning and coping.
- Identify high-risk situations for relapse.
- Attribute gains to patient's effort.
- Express sense of pride regarding the patient's new capacities.
- Express pride and satisfaction in the work together.

7.8.2 Termination Tactics

Action alternatives can be selected in the same way as in other phases of treatment.

Actively challenge tactical defences to keep focus on emotions related to ending therapy.

Identify and stay with the emotions. Link this with the central theme.

The relational focus may be activated by the anticipated loss of the therapist.

Collaborate with the patient to create a written summary of the therapy for patient to take away. Review what has been accomplished, what changes the patient has made, what is left to be done and what worked and what didn't.

Partir c'est mourir un peu!

7.8.3 Follow-Up and Outcome

To assess outcome, a follow-up meeting 1 year after termination may be helpful and also allow consolidation of gains. Ratings on outcome measures can be compared with results at the start and ending of therapy.

Key Points

- The goals of STPP are to enhance health and adaptive functioning.
- It is critical to establish a strong therapeutic alliance in the early phases of therapy.
- STPP involves three main phases: engagement, emotion processing and termination.
- Action alternatives can be selected based on choice point analysis.
- A relational focus is collaboratively developed in the early sessions.
- Getting past defences in order to process deep emotion is a strategic goal of STPP.
- Metaprocessing is a critically important therapeutic intervention.

References

1. Balint M, Ornstein P, Balint E. Focal psychotherapy. London: Tavistock Publications; 1972.
2. Gustafson JP. The complex secret of brief psychotherapy in the works of Malan and Balint. In: Gustafson JP, editor. The complex secret of brief psychotherapy. New York: W. W. Norton; 1986. p. 83–128.
3. Malan DH. Beyond interpretation: initial evaluation and technique in short-term dynamic psychotherapy. Part I. Int Journal Short Term Psychother. 1986;1:59–82.
4. Malan DH. Beyond interpretation: initial evaluation and technique in short-term dynamic psychotherapy. Part II. Int J Intensive Short Term Dyn Psychother. 1986;1:83–106.
5. Malan DH. The frontier of brief psychotherapy. New York: Plenum; 1976.
6. Mann J. Time-limited psychotherapy. Cambridge: Harvard University press; 1973.
7. Sifneos PE. Short-term dynamic psychotherapy: evaluation and technique. 2nd ed. New York: Plenum; 1987.
8. Luborsky L. Principles of psychoanalytic psychotherapy: a manual for supportive-expressive treatment. New York: Basic Books; 1984.
9. Fosha D. The transforming power of affect: a model for accelerated change. New York: Basic Books; 2000.
10. Leichsenring F, Schauenburg H. Empirically supported methods of short-term psychodynamic therapy in depression-towards an evidence-based unified protocol. J Affect Disord. 2014;169:128–43.
11. Lemma A, Target M, Fonagy P. Brief dynamic interpersonal therapy. Oxford Oxford University Press; 2011.
12. McCullogh L, Kuhn N, Andrews et al. Treating affect phobia a manual for short term dynamic psychotherapy. New York: Guilford press; 2003.
13. Abbass A. Reaching through resistance: advanced psychotherapy techniques. Kansas City: Seven leaves Press; 2015.
14. Coughlin P. Maximizing effectiveness in dynamic psychotherapy. New York: Routledge; 2017.
15. Kurtz S, Silverman J, Draper J. Teaching and learning communication skills in medicine. 2nd ed. Oxford: Radcliffe; 2005.
16. Shea SC. Psychiatric interviewing: the art of understanding. 2nd ed. Philadelphia WB Saunders; 1998.

17. Prenn N. Mind the gap: AEDP interventions translating attachment theory into clinical practice. J Psychother Integr. 2011;21(3):308–29.
18. Tauber L. Choice point analysis: formulation, strategy, intervention, and result in group process therapy and supervision. Int J Group Psychother. 1978;28(2):163–84.
19. Parkinson CN. The Economist. London. November 19, 1955.
20. Freud S. Analysis terminable and interminable. SE V.23 Hogarth; 1937.
21. Norcross JC, Greenberg RP, Swift JK. Do all therapists do that when saying goodbye? A study of commonalities in termination behaviors. Psychotherapy. 2017;54:66–75.

Chapter 8
Supervision: Applying Action Alternatives

8.1 Supervision Format

Tauber's method was to supervise small groups (Chap. 6) [1]. He felt a group of one supervisor and three supervisees was optimal. He used videotaped recordings of the students' sessions. During the supervision, the video is stopped at various points, and alternative actions are discussed. He utilized role-playing alternative interventions.

This would allow the supervisees to determine which was the preferred intervention.

I have used the basis of this approach with psychiatry residents over the past 6 years. I have used principally audio recordings of psychotherapy sessions. Video recording would be superior as it allows observation of non-verbal communication and cues.

I generally have met residents individually or in groups of two with or without one other supervisor who may be in training.

There are a large range of interventions. At any one moment, the therapist must consider 20 or more possible interventions. The reader is referred to Chap. 6 for a detailed description of choice point analysis and action alternatives. I have grouped therapist interventions into three priority sets of action alternatives:

A. Eppel, *Short-Term Psychodynamic Psychotherapy*, https://doi.org/10.1007/978-3-319-74995-2_8

- Relational and emotion-focused
- Defence
- Content

I will describe the supervision process of an audio-recorded session. The student gives a brief overview of the session. He may identify areas of uncertainty or difficulty.

A segment of the recording is played. The group members track the conversation paying attention to emotional cues: changes in voice tone, volume or prosody. At any point, any member of the supervisory group can ask for the recording to be stopped for clarifications.

The supervisor is alert to "choice point" cues from the patient that invite a response from the therapist. It is useful to refer to the triangle of defence to assess if the patient is in anxiety, defence or core emotion mode (Chap. 1).

8.2 Supervisory Questions to the Therapist

What were you feeling at this point in the interview?
Where did you feel the interview was going?
What action alternatives were you considering? Or humorously, "where are you going with this counsellor?"
What impact was the patient having on you in this segment?
What were you feeling then?

The supervisor can ask for the recording to be stopped and ask the group members in turn which action alternatives they might choose. This can be role-played with another member of the group taking the role of patient. The group can then discuss the reasons for the different choices. It is recognized that there is no one correct choice and that each intervention is an experiment. The nature of the patient's response determines the effectiveness of the intervention.

The supervisor should also point out opportunities where the therapist can link emotions and events to the selected relational focus.

8.2.1 Supervisory Questions About the Patient

What defences is the patient displaying at this point on the recording?
What feelings is he experiencing?
How did the patient appear to be viewing you?
Where on the triangle was the patient in that segment?

Transcript

Janet was a 44-year-old architect married for 16 years to a lawyer. She has no children.

Pt: One of my big stumbling blocks is taking on too much.

[00:00:55.11] Interviewer: Right.

Pt: And that yes...um...and I guess too because I'm just used to taking most of the responsibility for my stepfather.

[00:01:11.17] Interviewer: Mmm-hmm...

Pt: But my brother is busy and doesn't have as much time as I do to do stuff for her....yeah, but the self-sacrificing issue is interesting for me because I tend not to delegate well because for some reason I guess I just feel that I deserve to be overburdened...or that I'm used to being overburdened...

Action alternatives

Content	Affect-emotion	Transference	Rupture	Current relations
Past relations	Empathic	Silence	Validation	Defences
Metaprocess	Amplification	Portrayal	Relational focus	

[00:01:59.17] Interviewer: Is it something that you enjoy or something that no, you don't because self-sacrifice, it can mean many things to different people...

Pt: Yeah...yeah...I really have thought about that...if I enjoy it....if I get some kind of a....you know what I think it could partly be is like a...um....I had that concept in my head a minute ago and I can't think of it....it's like a moral advantage...I feel like I get the moral advantage...by taking most of the responsibility on myself...

Comment: Intellectual discussion here rather than going for emotion.

[00:02:52.10] Interviewer: How does that feel?

Pt: Well frustrating for one thing because I am....and resentful...I feel resentful...because um...yeah I do end up doing most of the work....and it's not like dad doesn't appreciate it but um....sometimes I get weary of being the go-to girl for everything...and that kind of also happens in other situations for me too....

Comment: Therapist goes for feelings but gets discussion about feelings.

Pt: And .....it would be good if I could get that under control....I think...

[00:03:40.20] Interviewer: We have talked a lot about the resentment piece and the frustration piece, and at the same time, when you call it a moral advantage...it kind of has a positive connotation as well...

Pt: Yeah...

[00:03:53.12] Interviewer: Is that correct?

Pt: Yeah...I feel morally superior...

[00:03:58.26] Interviewer: Mmm....

Pt: And I...I guess I hope that the other people who aren't taking as much responsibility are looked on as not doing their part....and.....um....yeah, I have to think about that one...it's a toughie....

Therapist using Set 3 intervention. Patient displays defences: intellectualizing, vagueness and isolation of affect. Going for the emotion of resentment might be a better choice.

Action alternatives

Content	Emotion	Transference	Rupture	Current relations
Past relations	Empathic	Silence	Validation	Defences
Metaprocess	Amplification	Portrayal	Relational focus	

[00:04:26.27] Interviewer: What does that feel like... to feel morally superior...what kind of emotions does that bring up for you?

Pt: Well kind of like....like I'll get a reward of some sort....I don't know what kind of reward I'd get but...

[00:04:53.19] Interviewer: Is there a particular feeling attached to it?

Pt: I'm trying to think of that....well I guess I just feel better about myself...

[00:05:06.05] Interviewer: Ok.

Pt: Um....I um....I guess I feel virtuous and...well I suppose and needed...um...and like I'm really doing this person some good...

[00:05:41.10] Interviewer: Mm-hmm...

Pt: But at the same time, if I do enough of it, I feel resentful...

[00:05:47.20] Interviewer: Mm-hmm....

Pt: So there's a balance to be struck....and...

[00:05:54.16] Interviewer: So on the one hand, it sounds like some positive kind of emotions attach to it... and then kind of, if you extend yourself too far, it's this resentment that comes up..

Comment: Going for feelings seems a good choice.

Action alternatives

Content	Emotion-emotion	Transference	Rupture	Current relations
Past relations	Empathic	Silence	Validation	Defences
Metaprocess	Amplification	Portrayal	Relational focus	

Pt: Yeah....I think at the core of it is that because I've always felt maligned....by doing all this stuff....all these good works...I am showing other people that I'm not so bad....

Pt: I think that's probably at the core of it...because yeah....um...

[00:06:43.19] Interviewer: It's very much in line it sounds like with kind of other things we've talked about like needing to please others...wanting to appear perfect... being kind of reasonable....they're all at the core...it almost seems like it's yourself being this performer that ….....you can't just be yourself...

Pt: Yeah....um....I feel I'm vindicating myself....

[00:07:17.04] Interviewer: Mmm-hmm..

Pt: Yes, by appearing...by being indispensable...

[00:07:23.08] Interviewer: Mm-hmm...

Pt: And that's a very hard one to get over....I think that's at the core of a lot of my issues is just the feeling of.....of being like I said, maligned...

[00:07:42.14] Interviewer: Mm-hmm...

Comment: The therapist chooses to go with relational focus, the need to please others because of a sense of self as worthless.

Pt: And that others don't have a good opinion of me and trying to deal with past issues where I felt worthless and persecuted and...

[00:08:00.05] Interviewer: Well you've carried that with you for some time....

Pt: Mmm-hmmm...

Action alternatives

Content	Emotion	Transference	Rupture	Current relations
Past relations	Empathic	Silence	Validation	Defences
Metaprocess	Amplification	Portrayal	Relational focus	

[00:08:03.27] Interviewer: Starting within your childhood...where it was always this proving yourself to your father...

Pt: Yeah....right.

[00:08:12.24] Interviewer: And then at school, that being the same and moving forward as well...

Pt: Mmm-hmmm....yeah....and I didn't know before I started therapy how really deep that problem is....

[00:08:30.28] Interviewer: Mmm-hmm..

Pt: I didn't really look at that issue in particular very closely I guess...I knew I had a problem there but I didn't know how pervasive....how serious it is....because it really...is the catalyst for a lot of my actions...yeah....

Comment: *Therapist connects relational focus to past relationships.*

Action alternatives

Content	Emotion	Transference	Rupture	Current relations
Past relations	Empathic	Silence	Validation	Defences
Metaprocess	Amplification	Portrayal	Relational focus	

[00:08:55.26] Interviewer: How does it feel to recognize that?

Pt: It feels some...it feels like....I'm sort of relieved... relief...a bit of relief because I knew I had a problem there...in that department....

[00:09:25.02] Interviewer: Mmm-hmm...

Pt: But how much of a problem, I had no idea...and so I would just think to myself...well my problems are very small compared to other people's problems and they're not really worth a lot of examination and....and anybody going to any trouble to help me figure them out and um...yeah kind of making light of them and that kind of thing, but no really I guess I feel relief in that it's a serious problem that I have right there in that instance, and uh....it is worth investigating...in fact, it's very important to investigate it....yeah...

Comment: Could go with transference "anybody going to any trouble…" is directed to the therapist.

[00:10:24.18] Interviewer: That's quite a big step.

Pt: Yes...I guess so....I would like to know ways to deal with it....to improve my self-image in that area... because I think a lot of my behaviour would...and a lot of my attitudes would um....could change if I knew that deep down I didn't deserve to be given a hard time.... yeah...and I didn't have to prove to people that I'm a good person....yeah....

[00:11:11.16] Interviewer: Well certainly I think you've made a lot of personal progress in discovering what's behind your actions and the way you interact with people and the patterns that you've had through your life....so you've made a lot of progress that way..... and you're right...now, the question is what do we do with this information...where do we go from here?

Comment: Too much of an intellectual discussion. One alternative would be going for feelings about being given a hard time.

Action alternatives

Content	Emotion	Transference	Rupture	Current relations
Past relations	Empathic	Silence	Validation	Defences
Metaprocess	Amplification	Portrayal	Relational focus	

Pt: Yes.

[00:11:36.22] Interviewer: When I ask that....what comes up for you?

Pt: Um...well first I'm glad you're suggesting another step ....to take another look at it from another angle... and...cause I think some kind of action has to be taken on it....yes....I welcome some additional attention to that matter....I do, yeah....I can't think of any better way to describe it....

[00:12:30.13] Interviewer: Well it sounds like it rings very true for you that you feel like you know....you'd like to initiate some sort of change in your life from this point on....

Comment: There is a misattunement here. The therapist is talking about changes based on the therapy so far. The patient is talking about a different form of therapy – CBT.

Pt: Yeah.

[00:12:39.08] Interviewer: I guess my question is.... what kinds of changes have you thought of or what kinds of things maybe has come up for you in thinking about this?

Pt: Well I guess the only one I can really think of that I've heard is effective ...and I'm sure there are lots of other ways to look at it and deal with it that are just as effective would be cognitive therapy....and um...when I've been reading this book that I have...it has a bunch of exercises and things to do that are...sound to me to be very rational....it's a really rational way to approach things, I think....

[00:13:28.04] Interviewer: I can see...I can hear where you're coming from but I do wonder if part of....I guess I'm curious as to why maybe you're own ideas haven't come up about how to change things in your life, given the insight that you've gotten, and I wonder if it's because you're still kind of looking at other people to give you direction...you're still feeling...

Pt: Yeah perhaps...

[00:13:59.10] Interviewer: Maybe in that self-doubting role...

Pt: Yeah...yup....perhaps...I think it's maybe cause it's....maybe the only behavioural therapy really that I've looked into with any detail....I think...for instance, I'm really interested in I guess it's Jungian-type therapy where you investigate different archetypes...is that right?

[00:14:29.27] Interviewer: Well I guess I'm just curious you know....have you got any ideas...outside of any kind of formal therapy or any kind of...?

Pt: Yeah...

[00:14:49.06] Interviewer: Because my sense is that you've been in this role of pleasing others and doing things for others...so what are you going to do about it now?

Comment: Alternative action is to explore feeling. "What do you feel when you reflect on always pleasing others?"

Pt: Definitely you've been telling me too....to take it easier on myself so that's where I'd have to start...that's a good place to start...and....that can have many different ways of expressing itself, for instance, you know let up on the perfectionism....and um.....things don't have to be so perfect and running like a top all the time...and if other people have issues with that, it's their problem....

[00:15:45.01] Interviewer: Mmm-hmmm...

Pt: For example, I guess I try to do too much in 1 day, and if I go overboard on one particular task and spend too much time on it or too much energy on it...then it really puts me behind doing all the other things

....and then I think to myself...and why do you feel like that? And it's because I've been knocking myself out all day to get all this stuff done that would please a lot of other people and it's perfectionism....yeah...

Comment: Intellectual defences. Therapist goes along.

[00:18:05.25] Interviewer: How could that be different I wonder?

Pt: Mm-hmm.....(chuckles)...yeah that's a hard one... that's a really hard one because....I'm not saying it's insurmountable...I think I'll have to be creative in dealing with that one...because I think a lot of it has to do with the fact that I am creative....and so I have a lot of ideas about what I want to do every day....and...I sort of set myself too many tasks and it's out of sheer enthusiasm usually...

[00:19:04.08] Interviewer: Ok...

Pt: Yeah...that I just want to do these things and I sort of feel an impetus to do it too....and uh....I think I have to curb my enthusiasm...yeah..

[00:19:27.15] Interviewer: I'm just curious...cause I kind of pushed you there a little bit ...because you gave me the answer of you know maybe cognitive behavioural therapy and I really kind of tried to push you in a different direction....what came up for you when I did that?

Pt: Well I guess I get the vibe really that cognitive therapy isn't really particularly on the menu....

Comment: Therapist now switches to address the transference and metaprocessing.

[00:19:58.14] Interviewer: But what's the feeling that you got when I did that?

Pt: Um....my feeling about it...um I guess.....I guess a bit dismayed...but um...I yeah....I uh...but curious about other things I could be doing...

[00:20:31.22] Interviewer: So tell me about feeling dismayed when I did that or....

Pt: Um....

[00:20:49.05] Interviewer: What did that feel like?

Pt: I guess because it's...yeah...I suppose it's the only form of therapy that I've been really examining....

[00:20:58.22] Interviewer: Mm-hmm...

Pt: Um closely and uh....

[00:21:04.03] Interviewer: And so what's the emotion that came when I kind of....pushed you in a different direction?

Pt: Oh um....well, a little frustrated...

[00:21:15.18] Interviewer: Mm-hmm..

Pt: Yeah...but I guess it's.....yeah...just a little frustrated...

[00:21:23.17] Interviewer: Tell me about that frustration....

Pt: Well I think it's....it...well I guess it's something that I think could possibly do me some good isn't particularly like I was saying, on the menu....(chuckles).... or isn't recommended...I guess I just kind of feel a little bit um....uninformed perhaps...I feel like....uh....that my idea isn't...acceptable...yeah I guess and um....

[00:22:16.18] Interviewer: I wonder what stopped you from voicing that in the moment?

Pt: I guess cause I don't really think about...yeah, I don't really think about my objections....or my feelings about things...I think I tend to take the ....a cooperator role and...not argue and try to adapt...

[00:22:45.22] Interviewer: Mm-hmm...

Pt: To the new tack....and um....

Comment: Therapist is trying to access emotion but is running into tactical defences. Some defence work might help: "I notice that when I try get in touch with your emotions you move to a factual discussion......."

[00:22:54.17] Interviewer: That's the sense that I got as well kind of.....when we had that interaction is this....I wonder if it's similar to how you might be kind of with your husband....

Pt: Yeah, sure....

[00:23:08.24] Interviewer: You know, with your friends...with other people in your life and maybe how you were with your father...I don't know if that rings...

Comment: Therapist links transference to current relationships, husband and friends.

Pt: Yeah..

[00:23:18.04] Interviewer: Rings true?

Pt: Yes...yeah, a lot of times, I have to settle for what other people want...and um....a lot of the times...you know how they say be true to yourself?

[00:23:32.15] Interviewer: Mm-hmm...

Pt: I'm not true to myself and I don't get what I want....out of situation or an experience because I've been too accommodating to others and....yeah and I feel resentful and frustrated...

Comment: Lots of resentment here. Better option is to go for the anger.

[00:23:52.02] Interviewer: Mm-hmm....

Pt: Um....and that's not to say really that other people's plans and ideas don't have merit...I guess I just...I think I just think of it in terms of well what would happen if we did this?

[00:24:13.04] Interviewer: Mm-hmm...

Pt: And sometimes I think....with some other people...um, they have to have their own way or it's the highway, and....they always....I'm not saying you in particular but other experience I've had with other people...you basically have to go along with them or they don't want anything to do with you, and....I found myself in with quite a few people like that...

Comment: Time to explore the anger.

[00:24:44.03] Interviewer: And how interesting that this played out even here...

Pt: Yeah...yes...well I think in the past I had mentioned cognitive therapy, and um...I think because it was quite early on, like a few months ago....really perhaps it was a little premature to mention it or to be talking about it....so I didn't really get a particular warm fuzzy feeling from you about it...

[00:25:19.12] Interviewer: Mmm.

Pt: I don't know if something like this could be up for discussion at this point in time perhaps...

[00:25:26.02] Interviewer: Mm-hmm.....

Pt: But certainly I'm open to other suggestions as well....

Action alternatives

Content	Emotion	Transference	Rupture	Current relations
Past relations	Empathic	Silence	Validation	Defences
Metaprocess	Amplification	Portrayal	Relational focus	

[00:25:32.26] Interviewer: Mm-hmm...I guess I'm more curious just about the interaction that we had.... you know, whether it's cognitive...the subject aside...I mean certainly we can talk about the role of cognitive behavioural therapy...I just find it so interesting that... you know this feeling of being....maybe...um...you know, not being able to voice your own opinion...even in a setting where we're here...

Pt: Yeah..

[00:26:10.12] Interviewer: That this pattern is playing out too...

Pt: Yeah...um yes...I think I tend to see almost everybody else as superior to me....and um...you know, they know more than me, or they're better educated than or they have more status than me, or...everybody seems to have some advantage over me in my mind....and I have to...defer to them..

[00:26:58.01] Interviewer: Mm-hmm....

Pt: And especially professionals...like in the medical profession or....or teachers or the accountant or the people at the bank or whoever...yeah....that I think I've mentioned...I always feel at a disadvantage with just about everybody...yes....I, just as ..an aside I guess one of the issues I had when my step dad was...I had to take him to the hospital ..the doctor gave me such a hard time and he kept coming at me with all of his...you know that in the hospital you have to basically get in line and wait your turn and we don't do this here, we don't do that there....and um....and it was all about rule...about the rules. I had to be...defiant

I really felt it much easier to kind of....tell like...stick to my guns about what we wanted...and um...I felt like a different person...

[00:31:01.07] Interviewer: Mm-hmm...

Comment: Strong relational and transference themes inviting exploration.

Pt: But I think it shook me to my core...that I had to behave that way towards authority... and I often think if it had been a different doctor.....I don't know if I would've stood up to him.

[00:31:34.10] Interviewer: So what was it like to stand up to the doctor?

Pt: Yeah, I felt like I was being a real pain.

[00:31:44.25] Interviewer: Hmm....

Pt: And giving and yeah, I felt like....I was really being a monster....

[00:32:25.18] Interviewer: Mm-hmm...

Pt: But I knew that I just couldn't let my stepfather be treated like this....

[00:32:43.03] Interviewer: How was it for you to tell me that you were feeling frustrated when I kind of maybe moved the topic away from cognitive behavioural therapy...how was it like for you to express that you were frustrated?

Pt: Well I do feel like I'm being difficult and um...that I'm yeah like I'm being cheeky and actually a little...I had a little glimmer of like the feeling I get standing up to my dad...

[00:33:23.22] Interviewer: Hmmm....

Pt: Like I'm not allowed...I'm absolutely not allowed to express...to show my opposition....

[00:33:33.01] Interviewer: Hmm...

Pt: Yeah....yes, and I'm being um....oh...antagonistic... yeah....mm-hmmm.....

[00:34:13.23] Interviewer: It sounds like any kind of expression of your own opinion leads you to feel that way.

Pt: Yes....that's right...

[00:34:27.21] Interviewer: Hmm....

Pt: Yeah...I'd say within a lot of...in most situations, my opinion is either greeted with....is dismissed....like outright dismissed or treated with disdain or ignored...

[00:34:59.12] Interviewer: And do you think I did that?

Comment: Therapist does a stellar job of addressing the transference.

Pt: Well I would hope you didn't have a....like a....I didn't think you were being mean about it (chuckles)...I uh....

[00:35:29.18] Interviewer: You laughed there a little bit...

Pt: Yeah....I couldn't find any better way to describe it....um yeah I didn't think your motivation to change tack was negative...I think just because in your role as the professional in the...in the um....the professional in this situation, I guess I just take it to mean to think that you know best and that I have to um...that uh....I have to to....I have to trust you so...

[00:36:30.10] Interviewer: If you did feel like I dismissed you or ignored you, would you feel comfortable saying that?

Pt: I think if you....no I wouldn't...no....

[00:36:50.16] Interviewer: Ok.

Pt: No...but I ....perhaps if you had behaved differently and I....had cause to feel offended....I wouldn't have told you no that I was offended....

[00:37:10.10] Interviewer: There was a twinge of that though...is my thought...that this pattern of feeling like your ideas are dismissed or...do you think that that's true....that that same feeling came up with me as it has come up with other people?

Pt: Perhaps to a very small degree...

[00:37:37.03] Interviewer: Mm-hmm..

Pt: Um....yeah...perhaps...maybe if you were...let's say we were just friends chatting...

[00:37:54.16] Interviewer: Mm-hmm...

Pt: Um...yeah, maybe I'd feel more irritated by it than I would if you are a professional...

[00:38:11.13] Interviewer: Mm-hmm..

Pt: It's all within the context for me you know of the situation and the relationship and the....yeah..it's a lot about power balance....yeah cause I always feel everybody else has way more power than I do, especially doctors (chuckles)....and yeah...

[00:38:41.09] Interviewer: I get the sense that's one element of it...and the other element is...at least in my sense of things is that in many of your relationships... that it's very hard to vocalize your own opinion and you are compliant and that leads to some negative feelings.

Pt: Yes...yeah...really...yes exactly...yeah and um.... yes, and it taints the relationship for me with a lot of people, and that I can't be real with them....and it makes the relationship very unequal...

Comment: Excellent transference work and links to other relationships.

[00:39:48.19] Interviewer: Mm-hmmm...

Pt: Um...mm-hmm..

[00:39:58.15] Interviewer: So I guess in this case I wonder you know....I wonder, given that now we're exploring that a little bit and maybe talking about some of the feelings that were behind...when we talked about cognitive behavioural therapy or didn't talk about cognitive behavioural therapy....what could you change or what could be different in our conversation that.... maybe would've led to...

Pt: Well I think I could've been a little more persistent...

[00:40:36.09] Interviewer: Mmmm...and what could you have said?

Pt: I think I'd first of all want to know ...why you seem hesitant to go in that direction....to examine that direction...

[00:40:56.23] Interviewer: Mm-hmm...so we can even do this now...as an exercise and also as a way to kind of....for me to give some information as well...so I think it's also interesting....that...the interpretation is hesitation about exploring cognitive behavioural therapy..... you seem to have a lot of interest in it...I think the reason why I tried to shift gears is to see if you feel confident in your own abilities to try to change things as opposed to....pursuing another therapy, for example...., because I have noticed that pattern for you, and you may disagree with that but you can tell me what you think.

Pt: Yeah...

Comment: Therapist is metaprocessing.

[00:41:59.03] Interviewer: Rather than feeling confident in your own ability ....is thinking oh maybe cognitive behavioural therapy will help me...maybe this therapy will help...maybe someone else can help me as opposed to yourself helping yourself...and that's where I was trying to shift the direction...not so much that that's a bad therapy or we shouldn't consider it...... but, at the same time, wondering if you feel empowered in your own self in terms of change without particularly looking for more therapy.

Pt: Looking to something outside of myself...yes....

[00:42:44.22] Interviewer: Yeah...similarly...

Pt: Yeah..

[00:43:09.25] Interviewer: And so I guess my goal or hope was to shift some of that external focus into something more that you can internalize...if that makes sense...

Pt: Yes, I guess...I'd like to examine that closer... yeah...and then...find ways that I could do that more..

[00:43:35.02] Interviewer: And I do apologize if it seemed more like I was hesitating to go to the cognitive behavioural therapy part....I think what I wanted to do was to try to focus maybe on what you feel you might be able to do for yourself as well...but I do apologize if it came off to be that way...

Pt: Oh, that's quite alright...(chuckles)...yeah, uh... yes, I'd be happy to examine ways I could find health within myself.....

Comment: Therapist apologizes which has the effect of validating patient and counteracting her feelings about doctors being superior.

[00:48:12.21] Interviewer: Ok...how are you feeling right now...cause I know it's a lot to kind of....it's actually..

Pt: I feel a little tired (chuckles).

[00:48:19.10] Interviewer: It is work to talk about how our interactions are in the moment...it can actually be a very tiring...

Pt: Mmm-hmm...yes....yes....well I guess I feel a little awkward..

[00:48:35.02] Interviewer: Mm-hmm..

Pt: Yeah...um...I guess cause I'm not used to being real with people...

[00:48:41.29] Interviewer: Mmm....

Pt: And the roof hasn't caved in (chuckles)...that's nice....(chuckles).

[00:48:54.00] Interviewer: I know you say that jokingly...

Pt: Yeah..or you haven't stormed out of the office... saying, I'll never see you again and that kind of thing... the world hasn't come to an end so..

[00:49:07.06] Interviewer: Is that sometimes your fear....when you do kind of talk in...like you said, a real way or?

Pt: Yeah..with other people...with my friends or with my husband..I'm always afraid of inflaming people... yeah...and making them feel uncomfortable...and...and making them think ill of me and um...yeah...

[00:49:50.14] Interviewer: I could imagine it is actually quite different to say, for example, that you were frustrated or...to...it's a way of kind of being vulnerable or...or extending yourself in a very uncomfortable way..

Pt: Yes...yes...it almost makes me squirm inside...to feel like that...to be asking for what I want and being honest...to be honest with people...yeah cause a lot of fear comes up...and uh...yeah just a lot of fear...

Comment: Excellent relational work and metaprocessing.

[00:50:47.02] Interviewer: Mm-hmm....

Pt: I think a lot of the time I invest so much in a situation or a relationship that yeah..basically the whole thing is built on my fear that it's going to end if I'm not careful...

[00:51:14.16] Interviewer: Mm-hmm..

Pt: And that I could blow it by saying the wrong thing...

[00:51:22.00] Interviewer: Mm-hmm..

Pt: And that one misstep will destroy it all..yeah..

[00:51:30.13] Interviewer: So there's always this inhibition..

Pt: Yeah..that's right...

[00:51:35.28] Interviewer: Mm-hmm...

Pt: Perhaps that's why I have so very few outside relationships...outside the family..I've never really had a lot of friends at one time...and uh....there's really nobody that I've ever thought of as very close...that I could confide in...or be really real with...yeah...um....I've always kept people at arm's length when it comes to really telling them what I think and being real...

Comment: Patient displays good appreciation of relational themes.

[00:52:28.21] Interviewer: To me, it almost seems like, in a way, becomes second nature to be compliant all the time and maybe to not be "real".

Pt: Yes..

[00:52:45.02] Interviewer: Because even in our interaction I think it took a little bit of a pause to really... recognize that there was some frustration or...do you think that that was true or did you recognize it right away..but maybe didn't want to say anything or...

Pt: Hmm...yes, I guess I didn't...I recognize the pause...and..I was a little...you know, a little bit irritated by it...but I...I don't think it was something I really felt compelled, you know...to say anything about..

[00:53:47.13] Interviewer: Mm-hmm...and that's kind...that's kind of your natural tendency or...is that correct or?

Pt: Yeah..I guess...yeah......I really wasn't that... offended or anything by it...now...but even then... I won't say anything if it really seriously bothers me and offends me, and yeah, I won't say anything then either.

[00:54:32.23] Interviewer: Mm-hmm..

Comment: Therapist comes back to the transference to reinforce the themes.

8.3 Structured Assessment of Sessions

Many systems have been developed for assessing and coding process elements in therapy sessions. Leigh McCullough and colleagues at Harvard developed the Achievement of Therapeutic Objectives Scale [2, 3]. More than a decade of research has been undertaken with this scale. This has involved video recordings and analyses of therapy sessions. Kristin Osborn, currently director at the Harvard Medical School Psychotherapy Research Program, has continued McCullough's work and developed a therapist rating version of the ATOS [4, 5].

Both of these scales are used with video recordings of psychotherapy sessions. Ratings are made of 10 min segments of the recording.

Both the ATOS and ATOS Therapist are rated on a scale of 1 to 100.

The ATOS is an example of a scale that can be used to assess patient outcome along dimensions that are highly relevant to psychodynamic psychotherapy. This includes ratings of the patient's awareness of maladaptive patterns of thoughts, feelings and behaviours; the patient's ability to fully experience emotion; a rating of verbal and non-verbal indications of anxiety, guilt and shame; the ability to express thoughts, feelings, wishes and needs; and changes in sense of self and sense of others.

The ATOS scale is based on whether the patient is able to recognize their defences, whether they can experience and express emotion, and the level of the inhibitory emotions of anxiety, guilt and shame.

The ATOS Therapist scale was designed to assess how well the therapist uses interventions to help the patient achieve the therapeutic objectives. It also serves as a fidelity measure to a particular model of psychotherapy. From a supervisory point of view, the ATOS Therapist can be used to evaluate the therapist's use of specific interventions.

The ATOS Therapist includes ratings of the therapist's awareness and insight into the patient's maladaptive patterns (defences) and his ability to communicate this to the patient, whether the therapist is able to increase the patient's motivation to give up these maladaptive patterns; whether the therapist helps the patient to experience adaptive emotions and helps to regulate feelings of anxiety, guilt and shame. Does the therapist assist the patient in improving his image of himself and image of others?

Training is available for the use of these scales through the affect phobia therapy website [3, 4].

8.3.1 *Verona Coding of Emotional Sequences: VR-CoDES*

A completely generic and widely researched coding system has been developed by the Verona Network on Sequence Analysis. The aim of this project is to develop a coding system that can capture how healthcare providers respond to patients' emotions [6, 7]. This system has been designed to apply to general healthcare. and creates a common language and coding system for research purposes. It may well be applicable to psychotherapy research given its generic language and clearly operationalized procedures.

The method is based on the study of sequences of patient cues and healthcare provider responses. It classifies the way patients express emotion in terms of cues and concerns. A cue is a verbal or non-verbal "hint" that points to an underlying emotion. A concern is defined as a clearly stated disturbing emotion, e.g. *I am sad.*

The VR-CoDES also provide a descriptive classification of the providers' responses. This system is operationally defined. Responses are classified based on whether they explicitly refer to the patient's cue or concern using wording that links the two and, secondly, whether the healthcare provider provides space or reduces the space that facilitates further disclosure of the cue or concern

Explicit responses require the provider to remain focused on and interested in the patient's expressions. The provider must acknowledge explicitly the patient's emotional signals and respond empathically.

The provider can allow more space for the patient to communicate by encouraging and affirming statements, seeking clarification and specifically naming the emotion. Other response include active questioning about the emotional content or the use of silence.

Conversely giving premature advice, minimizing or devaluing what the patient has said and devaluing or dismissing the patient's emotions can lead to "reducing space" and shutting down the interview.

Key Points

- Choice point analysis is an excellent tool for psychotherapy supervision.
- It requires video or audio recordings of psychotherapy sessions.
- Supervisors and peers can review the recordings and identify points for intervention.
- The supervisory group can discuss alternative actions and decide which may be best to facilitate the therapy process and goals.
- The ATOS Therapist and the VR-CoDES are assessment systems that have potential for more widespread use in supervision.

8.4 Conclusion

Psychotherapy supervision is greatly facilitated by the use of choice point analysis and selection of action alternatives. This requires video or audio recordings in a setting of group or individual supervision. This method can be used for all levels of trainees in psychiatry, psychology, social work and related therapy professions.

Areas for future enhancement of this process include the utilization of instruments such as the ATOS Therapist and Verona Coding of Emotional Sequences. These types of measures could also facilitate psychotherapy process research.

References

1. Tauber L. Choice point analysis-formulation, strategy, intervention, and result in group process therapy and supervision. Int J group Psychotherapy. 1978;28:163–84.

2. McCullogh L, Kuhn N, Andrews, et al. Treating affect phobia a manual for short term dynamic psychotherapy. New York: Guilford press; 2003.
3. McCullogh L. Achievement of Therapeutic Objectives Scale. The Psychotherapy Research Program Harvard Medical School. http://www.affectphobiatherapy.com/research-scales/.
4. Osborn K. ATOS therapist 20 point brief rating guides. The Psychotherapy Research Program Harvard Medical School http://www.affectphobiatherapy.com/research-scales/.
5. Donovan JM, Osborn KA, Rice S. Paraverbal communication in psychotherapy: beyond the words. New York: Rowman & Littlefield; 2017.
6. Piccolo LD, Finset A, Mellblom AV, Figueiredo-Braga M, Korsvold L, Zhou Y, Zimmermann C, Humphris G. Verona Coding Definitions of Emotional Sequences (VR-CoDES): conceptual framework and future directions. Patient Educ Couns. 2017;100(12):2303–11. https://doi.org/10.1016/j.pec.2017.06.026. Epub 2017 Jun 21.
7. Del Piccolo L. VR-CoDES and patient-centeredness. The intersection points between a measure and a concept. Patient Educ Couns. 2017;100(11):2135–7. https://doi.org/10.1016/j.pec.2017.05.007. Epub 2017 May 5. PubMed PMID: 28610822.

Chapter 9
Psychodynamically Informed Clinical Practice for Non-Psychotherapists

9.1 Background

Not all clinicians are in a position to practice psychotherapy. Other work demands may preempt such opportunities. Institutional and funding policies may also limit job roles.

For healthcare practitioners in primary care, there may be no time to spend in formal psychotherapy. Nevertheless the insights and interventions that are part of psychodynamic psychotherapy can be enormously helpful in all areas of healthcare.

The psychodynamic framework offers a way to understand human behaviour, emotions and relationships. All of these dimensions impact on the experience of illness. The same variables come into play in the relationships between patients and physicians, nurses, psychologists, social workers and other healthcare workers.

This has relevance in all clinical settings whether outpatient, inpatient or community locations. Admission to the hospital places unique stresses on the individual's capacity to cope. There is the loss of autonomy, and forced dependency and assaults on bodily and psychological integrity.

A. Eppel, *Short-Term Psychodynamic Psychotherapy*,
https://doi.org/10.1007/978-3-319-74995-2_9

The patient's defences may be stretched, and his/her ability to regulate emotions may be impaired. If the healthcare team reacts on the surface without understanding the underlying dynamics, conflict or even rupture in the relationship between patient and the team may occur.

9.2 The Therapeutic Alliance and Attachment

Just as in formal psychotherapy, the therapeutic alliance is strongly correlated with medication treatment outcomes [1, 2].

Attachment style is a factor in all relationships and will influence the therapeutic alliance [3–7]. During the course of child development, internal working models are created (Chap. 2 this volume). These internal working models determine the patient's implicit expectations about intimate and caregiving relationships.

Patients with secure attachment have a positive expectation of help. They are able to trust healthcare providers. Patients with dismissing attachment style display relational patterns in which there is an implicit expectation of rejection. They have difficulty asking for help as this will make them vulnerable to rejection. They avoid closeness and have an overly developed preference for self-reliance. They may minimize the severity of their symptoms and not seek help. Patients with preoccupied attachment may exhibit greater emotional dysregulation and anxiety. They have a stronger need to be in contact with the physician. Their expression of symptoms has a transactional significance based on the underlying need for more secure attachments.

Maunder and colleagues studied 119 individuals who completed an online survey. The results demonstrated the influence of secure or insecure attachment on the patient's experience with healthcare providers [3]. In this study three factors were identified reflecting the patient's experience of the healthcare provider.

- The first factor named "support" is derived from patients who experienced the healthcare provider as safe and supportive.
- The second factor was termed "averse" and was associated with patients who experienced the provider as aversive.
- The third factor "want" reflected patient's desires to have more and closer contact with the provider.

The second and third factors correlated with attachment insecurity as measured by the Experience in Close Relationships questionnaire [3].

In a study of 165 patients and 26 emergency room physicians [4], patients with higher attachment anxiety and avoidance were perceived by the physician as more difficult. In this case the term "difficult" is used not in terms of diagnostic or treatment difficulty but in terms of the interaction between the patient and the physician. 98% of patients with secure attachment were not perceived as difficult. 17% of patients with preoccupied attachment were experienced as difficult. A further 19% of those with dismissing attachment and 39% of those with fearful attachment were felt to be "difficult" (Fig. 9.1).

The effect of patient attachment style has also been studied in the care of people with chronic illness and diabetes [5, 6]. In a study of 167 patients who had coronary artery bypass graft surgery, Kidd et al. [7] found that attachment anxiety was associated with both longer lengths of stay and higher plasma levels of interleukin 6.

9.3 Medication as Object and Psychodynamic Psychopharmacology

Transference and therapeutic alliance are just as fundamental in the practice of psychopharmacology as they are in the practice of psychotherapy The patient's attachment style and relationship templates will colour the interaction with healthcare providers. A patient's response to the prescription or indeed lack of prescription of medications will be influenced

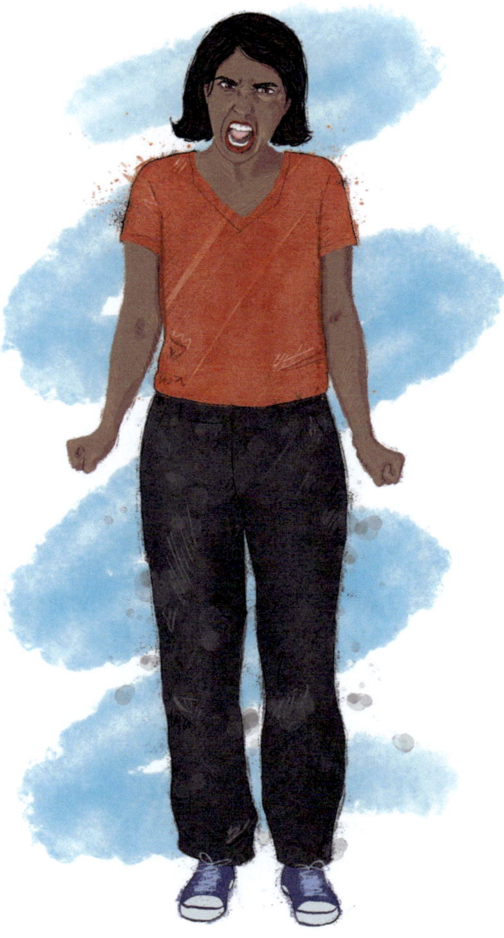

FIGURE 9.1 Anger. (Illustrations by Molly Ferguson www.MollyFergusonArt.com)

by their unconscious transference feelings and internal working models.

Adele Tutter has described how medication can be related to as if it were an object/person [8]. An individual's response to treatment interventions whether it is the administration of medication, a surgical procedure or an investigation is based on their habitual self-representation/self-image and their expectancies of the other person along with associated emotions.

At an unconscious level, the medication is a transitional object, a symbol or stand-in for the healthcare provider. Attributes of the healthcare provider may unconsciously be linked to the medication. The medication may be felt to represent the healthcare provider's compassion and concern. Conversely it might represent an attempt to intrude, invade, control or influence the patient's behaviour or personality. Medication is a powerful symbol because it is something external that is taken into the body [9].

Medication also conveys the message that the patient is defective or ill; this leads to the faulty logic that if the medication is stopped, the illness no longer exists.

The patient may feel submissive or dependent in acquiescing to taking medication.

Without a psychodynamic framework, the patient's behaviour is frequently misunderstood and the healthcare provider's response misattuned.

The offering of medications may trigger feelings about attachment figures who are obliged to take medications, were very ill or have used medications.

The giving of a diagnosis can provoke resistance because of the linkage to a significant figure who had this diagnosis. This is "guilt by association" but may lead to the patient refusing treatment or being nonadherent to treatment.

The offering of medication can be perceived as dismissal or rejection, a brushoff. Alternatively providing a prescription may mean to the patient that the prescriber is understanding, empathic and caring.

Conversely a failure to offer medication can be perceived as dismissal or rejection depending on the individual patient: "*you don't take me seriously*".

The same principles apply in maintaining a good therapeutic alliance (Chap. 5).

Krupnick [1] and Meyer [2] demonstrated that the quality of the therapeutic alliance contributed very significantly to positive outcome in treatment with antidepressants.

Adherence to or "compliance with a prescriber's prescription" is influenced by dynamic factors: the therapeutic alliance, transference based on being told to "comply" and unconscious unwanted identification with family members who have the same condition.

9.4 Relational Pattern

An individual's relational patterns will inevitably affect their responses and reactions. This applies not only to medication but to other treatment or social interventions made by healthcare or social service providers.

For example, individuals who view themselves as unworthy may be compliant on the surface because of fears they will be rejected or abandoned. Those who have a self-representation of failure may seek to reassure the prescriber that they are doing well even if this is not the case. Those with a self-view of unworthiness or not deserving of love may attempt to please the prescriber in the hope of being accepted.

Those who feel they are deserving of punishment or mistreatment may persist when the treatment causes uncomfortable side effects without reporting them.

More complex patterns involve unconscious needs to reject the physician's generosity or to mistrust based on prior experiences of abuse and betrayal.

Some patients may resist the necessary feelings of dependency of having to visit the physician for repeat prescriptions. Others may feel that medication is "a crutch" (although if your leg is broken you may need a crutch).

9.5 History Taking

Focusing on dynamic factors can result in more valid elicitation of information as well as promoting a more solid therapeutic alliance. This is critical for diagnosis and effective treatment of patients with all types of illnesses.

Time spent on attending to the interpersonal and dynamic characteristics of patients will pay off in the long run by establishing a better alliance and yielding better quality information.

Conversely a reliance on checklists and a barrage of closed-ended questions will yield poor quality responses, increase patient anxiety and lower quality of information provided.

Healthcare providers should use the dynamic interventions of empathy, attunement and validation rather than directive, authoritarian and rapid fire questioning.

Healthcare providers trained to recognize recurrent interpersonal patterns, and transference expectations can intervene more accurately and appropriately responding to patients needs. Similarly conflict in the provider-patient relationship may reflect transference reenactments and insecure attachment patterns.

9.6 Michael Balint

Balint was a pioneer in emphasizing the usefulness of the psychotherapeutic approach in general practice [10]. Balint crystallized his ideas in his concept of the physician as "drug." This contains the idea of the doctor presenting himself to the patient in a certain manner. Patients present with a hidden agenda; many of the real transactions are occurring covertly or unconsciously. There is an unconscious negotiation and implicit testing of the waters.

Balint described the patient's presenting problems as an offering and seeking a healing response. Balint recognized that physicians have difficulty dealing with the patient's psychological problems due to conventional expectations of the physician-patient interaction. Teaching psychotherapeutic skills involves helping clinicians become aware of their own emotional responses.

9.7 Ultrashort-Term Psychotherapy

Psychiatrists, physicians, psychologists and others who have time limits that preclude even short-term psychodynamic psychotherapy may be able to utilize intermittent sessions or ultrashort-term psychotherapy.

Donald Winnicott described ultrashort psychotherapeutic consultations consisting of 2–3 h sessions up to several months apart. Winnicott's goal was to elicit from the patient what was "worthwhile". He helped the patient to reveal what they felt was the worst and the best about themselves. Winnicott believed that we become ourselves "in the eyes of others". It follows therefore that we can shape our self-view by experiencing what others see in us [11].

This is a very profound statement and foreshadows a central tenet of the attachment approach to psychotherapy. Our self-identity is formed through our attachment relationships and is replayed and open to modification in our relationships with a therapist. It involves the feeling of being seen and being held in mind by another person.

Winnicott's therapeutic virtuosity was in accepting what the patient felt was "terrible" about himself and by listening without judgement to the things that the patient felt most ashamed and guilty about. Winnicott fostered a therapeutic setting in which the patient could "reveal" his deepest feelings of "badness".

Winnicott's genius was then to find a time in the patient's life when he felt "worthwhile". He worked this through by attending to the most negative feelings about the self and moving back and forth to what was most worthwhile [11]. The patient shares his fears and the therapist needs to admire what is worthwhile in the patient.

Winnicott felt it was important to identify and acknowledge inner feelings of destructiveness and in a complementary fashion to reach back to recover the goodness that was lost. This is based on his formulation that loss leads to aggressive and destructive emotions in an attempt to alter the external environment. In Winnicott's words this is an attempt "to force the environment to take notice".

The therapist's task is to acknowledge the loss and disappointment, to face the angry destructiveness and to survive: "Accept what is terrible and reach for the worthwhile". *I accept you despite all the bad things which are part of you (and I am not destroyed)* [11].

9.8 Thomas Main

A familiarity with the principles of short-term psychodynamic psychotherapy can help healthcare workers recognize the impact of their own feelings on their interactions with patients. Each of us brings with us our own internal working models and expectancies. These will shape our feelings towards and responses to patients. Working with individuals who are very ill can trigger fears and threaten our own sense of security and identity.

In a magnificently insightful presentation at the Ontario Psychiatric Association Annual Meeting in Toronto published in 1977, Main elucidates a range of personal, administrative and institutional procedures that defend clinicians from the feelings they experience in encounters with patients [12].

Physicians are prone to the same feelings as the rest of humanity. When faced with psychiatric illness, death and dying or demanding treatment challenges, a physician may experience the rise of anxiety that triggers defensive responses. Main describes one such defence as a retreat into biological psychiatry. This puts the physician into the role of "an uninvolved observer"; the subjectivity of the patient becomes marginalized. Physicians and other healthcare professionals may exhibit the defences of isolation of affect, intellectualization, devaluation, reaction formation and humour.

Reaction formation may result in the physician undertaking overzealous and futile treatment endeavours. This can be motivated by the physician's own fears of death and dying.

An extreme but potentially lethal example of the impact of the clinicians own nonconscious feelings towards certain patients, is described in a classic article about countertransference hate towards suicidal patients [13]. While this may be shocking to some readers, it provides some profound insights into the therapist and clinicians' responses to alarming and demanding clinical encounters. Clinicians can be overwhelmed with anxiety and feelings of helplessness.

Patients may be objectified to avoid acknowledgement of their humanity. They may be labelled as a diagnosis rather than a person: "*the diabetic in room 246*". In psychiatry this objectification may be reinforced by our diagnostic systems which rely on external symptoms and signs.

Institutional procedures can also lead to the objectification of patients. Psychological distance is created which can protect the staff from the anxiety of having to feel the patient's distress. Hospital and clinic roles may be fragmented so that the patient is reduced from being a whole person to a series of functions divided among a multidisciplinary staff.

The antidote to these undesirable occurrences starts with self-awareness and understanding. Supervisory relationships, peer consultation and team meetings provide an opportunity for healthcare workers to come to grips with their responses to patients.

Key Points

- Knowledge of the concepts and principles of short-term psychodynamic psychotherapy can help general clinicians improve their interactions with patients.
- It is important for all healthcare providers to be aware of their own emotional reactions to patients.
- Clinicians should understand the institutional and personal defence mechanisms that protect them from experiencing anxiety and helplessness.
- These defences can lead to avoidance of necessary close encounters with patients.

References

1. Krupnick JL, Sotsky SM, Simmens S, Moyer J, Elkin I, Watkins J, Pilkonis PA. The role of the therapeutic alliance in psychotherapy and pharmacotherapy outcome: findings in the National Institute of Mental Health Treatment of Depression Collaborative Research Program. J Consult Clin Psychol. 1996;64(3):532–9.

2. Meyer B, Pilkonis PA, Krupnick JL, Egan MK, Simmens SJ, Sotsky SM. Treatment expectancies, patient alliance, and outcome: further analyses from the National Institute of Mental Health Treatment of Depression Collaborative Research Program. J Consult Clin Psychol. 2002;70(4):1051–5.
3. Maunder RG, Hunter JJ. Can patients be 'attached' to healthcare providers? An observational study to measure attachment phenomena in patient-provider relationships. BMJ Open. 2016;6:e011068. https://doi.org/10.1136/bmjopen-2016-011068.
4. Maunder RG, Panzerb A, Viljoenc M, Owenc J, Humanc S, Hunterd JJ. Physicians' difficulty with emergency department patients is related to patients' attachment style. Soc Sci Med. 2006;63(2):552–62.
5. Ciechanowski PS, Katon WJ, Russo JE, Walker EA. The patient provider relationship: attachment theory and adherence to treatment in diabetes. Am J Psychiatr. 2001;158:29–35.
6. Ciechanowski PS, Russo JE, Katon WJ, Korff MV, Simon GE, Lin EH, et al. The association of patient relationship style and outcomes in collaborative care treatment for depression in patients with diabetes. Med Care. 2006;44:283–91.
7. Kidd T, Poole L, Elizabeth Leigh E, Ronaldson A, Jahangiri M, Steptoe A. Attachment anxiety predicts IL-6 and length of hospital stay in coronary artery bypass graft surgery (CABG) patients. J Psychosom Res. 2014;77(2):155–7.
8. Tutter A. J Am Psychoanalytic Assoc. 2006 Summer;54(3):781–804.
9. Hahn RA. The nocebo phenomenon: concept, evidence, and implications for public health. Prev Med. 1997;26:607–11.
10. Balint M. The doctor, his patient and the illness. London: Pitman Med; 1957.
11. Winnicott D. Therapeutic consultations in child psychiatry. London: Hogarth Press; 1971.
12. Main TF. Traditional psychiatric defences against close encounter with patients. Can Psychiatr Assoc J. 1977;22:457–66.
13. Maltsberger JT, Buie DH. Countertransference hate in the treatment of suicidal patients. Arch Gen Psychiatry. 1974;30(5):625–33.

Index

A. Eppel, *Short-Term Psychodynamic Psychotherapy*,
https://doi.org/10.1007/978-3-319-74995-2

MIX
Papier aus verantwortungsvollen Quellen
Paper from responsible sources
FSC® C105338

If you have any concerns about our products,
you can contact us on
ProductSafety@springernature.com

In case Publisher is established outside the EU,
the EU authorized representative is:
Springer Nature Customer Service Center GmbH
Europaplatz 3, 69115 Heidelberg, Germany

Printed by Libri Plureos GmbH
in Hamburg, Germany